KNOW YOUR REAL RISK OF
HEART ATTACK?

HOW TO KNOW IF THE SINGLE BIGGEST KILLER IS LURKING INSIDE YOU AND WHAT TO DO ABOUT IT

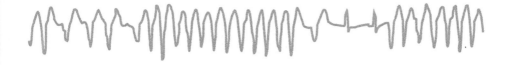

DR WARRICK BISHOP

KNOW YOUR REAL RISK OF
HEART ATTACK?

HOW TO KNOW IF THE SINGLE BIGGEST KILLER IS LURKING INSIDE YOU AND WHAT TO DO ABOUT IT

bringing the future into the present

This book is for you, if you:

- want to reduce your risk of a heart attack;
- have high cholesterol and are not sure about taking statins;
- suffer side-effects from statins;
- come from a family with 'bad' hearts;
- just want to know what's going on with your heart;
- want to know more about cardiac CT imaging;
- would enjoy an informative read about the main killer of our generation;
- believe prevention is better than cure, or
- are a doctor wanting more information about risk or need a book you can recommend to your patients.

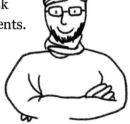

This book is also for you, if you have a heart.

Publisher's Note

The author and editors of this publication have made every effort to provide information that is accurate and complete as of the date of publication. Readers are advised not to rely on the information provided without consulting their own medical advisers. It is the responsibility of the reader's treating physician or specialist, who relies on experience and knowledge about the patient, to determine the condition of, and the best treatment for, the reader. The information contained in this publication is provided without warranty of any kind. The author and editors disclaim responsibility for any errors, mis-statements, typographical errors or omissions in this publication.

National Library of Australia Cataloguing-in-Publication entry

Author:	Bishop, Dr Warrick
Title:	Know Your Real Risk of Heart Attack?
ISBN:	
Subject:	Cardiac health care
Published:	Dr Warrick Bishop
Written with:	Penelope Edman
Cover design:	Doodlefish Web Design
Internal design:	Cathy McAuliffe Design
Illustrations:	Cathy McAuliffe Design

ISBN-10: 1986361322 (Amazon Paperback Print)

ISBN-13: 978-1986361323 (Amazon Paperback Print)

ISBN-10: 1642045705 (Hard Cover Print)

ISBN-13: 978-1642045703 (Hard Cover Print)

ASIN: B07BC9ZM8Q (Amazon Kindle)

ISBN: 9781370024193 (Smashwords)

Also available in Audiobook from

Amazon/Audible Audiobooks, Now Audiobooks.com, BookMate, Downpour, Hoopla, Hummingbird Media, Kobo, Libro.FM, Overdrive, StoryTel

*To my parents, Chris and Marie,
who taught me persistence, quality,
integrity and humility the best way
possible - by example.*

Contents

Foreword

Professor of Medicine, David Geffen School of Medicine, Harbor-UCLA Medical Center
Program Director and Director of Cardiac CT, Division of Cardiology, Harbor-UCLA Medical Center
Endowed Chair of Preventive Cardiology, Los Angeles Biomedical Research Institute

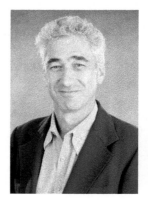

We have unprecedented opportunities to look earlier and safer into our coronary arteries. We have to remember that heart disease is the number one killer, of men and women, in the world. Ten times as many women will die of heart disease as breast cancer each year, yet we sometimes lose focus on the important aspects of our health. Warrick Bishop carefully and clearly outlines a path to better health, to longer life, and to improved outcomes. The CT scanner, with non-invasive methods to see the plaque building up in our pipes, will allow us to act earlier, when disease is reversible.

Too often in cardiology, I see patients when it is too late, either when they are dying or have already suffered massive heart damage. I know, that a simple heart scan, could have identified them ten-twenty years earlier, and allowed our effective heart treatments (both lifestyle and medications) to do their work and reverse the heart disease. The benefits of reading this book will only be limited by it's readership. It is so hard to find an accurate, easy to understand book, that is so applicable to almost all of us. If I can ask you to do one favor to save a life, it is to pass along this book to someone else who can act on it once you are done. The greatest gift would be to have more people have access to this important information. The more people who get the heart scan, the larger reductions in sudden cardiac death we will see. In the long-running war on heart disease, we are winning, and this book could help end it.

Matthew Budoff MD

Professor of Medicine, UCLA School of Medicine

Endowed Chair of Preventive Cardiology

About Matthew Budoff MD

Dr. Matthew Budoff is at the forefront of the medical community's efforts to develop early detection methods for cardiac disease, the number one cause of death in the U.S. Given that approximately 50 percent of U.S. heart disease victims learn of their illness by experiencing a sometimes fatal heart attack, Dr. Budoff has devoted much of his time over the past 25 years to advancing procedures that can help doctors identify cardiac patients early, and place them on a therapeutic path to prevent a heart attack.

Dr. Budoff works on at least 20 active medical research trials at any given time, and is a frequent lecturer on topics of cardiology at symposia, congresses and annual conferences on every continent. He has authored or co-authored over 800 research papers, seven books, and 45 book chapters.

Dr. Budoff has been listed among *America's and Los Angeles' Top Doctors* every year since 2005. In the past two years alone, Dr. Budoff has been honored with multiple awards recognizing his professional skills and accomplishments. Of particular note is his receipt of the Einstein Award for Scientific Achievement from the International Biographical Centre, Cambridge, U.K.; being named to the US News list of Top Doctors for 2011; and, most recently, named to "Worlds Most Influential Scientific Minds" in 2014. In 2015, he was awarded the Endowed Chair of Preventive Cardiology at his institution and the *Arthur S. Agatston Cardiovascular Disease Prevention Award*. In 2016, he was inducted into the European Union Academy of Sciences and honored with the prestigious Gold Medal Award by the Society of Cardiovascular Computed Tomography.

Dr. Budoff graduated *cum laude* from the University of California, Riverside. He graduated with distinction and a member of Alpha Omega Alpha from the George Washington University School of Medicine, in Washington, DC, then completed an internship and residency in internal medicine, and a fellowship in cardiology, at Harbor-UCLA Medical Center in Torrance, where he currently acts as Program Director for the Cardiology Fellowship and Director of Cardiac Computed Tomography.

Preface

If you're reading this, you can reasonably assume, despite my journalistic lifestyle and my cholesterol level, that I am still alive. My cardiologist, who is the author and publisher of this book, would not have prefaced a work on cardiac health with the thoughts of a dead patient. So I'm still here. That's the good news. Thanks, Doc!

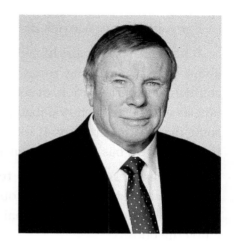

The bad news is, that in Australia, heart failure is the cause of more than 30 percent of deaths every year and most of these are due to coronary heart disease. This book confronts that stark reality in a readable, informative and practical way.

Are we, by diet and lifestyle, our own worst enemies? Or are we hapless victims of a cruelly indifferent genetic lottery? And the harder question: in either of those alternatives, what can we do about it?

In my work as a journalist I travel to some of the most remote parts of the world and it slowly occurred to me that Afghanistan or Antarctica would be inconvenient spots to suffer a heart attack. As you will learn from this book, the traditional medical evaluations of the state of the heart are often just highly educated guess work. Cardiologists admit you can pass a stress test one week and die the next. Because I needed to get to the heart of the matter, I wanted to know what was going on in there.

Your author, and my cardiologist, Warrick Bishop, is a lean and determined-looking man whose shaven head and athletic fitness bring to mind Vladimir Putin, without the unhappy associations. Indeed, what drew me to Dr Bishop was that he specialises in looking inside the working heart.

Using non-invasive imaging technology, he sees inside our coronary arteriesto determine just how rusted and encrusted the pipes have become.

For you and me, Warrick Bishop's picture is worth a thousand words.

It's our hearts, the very lifeblood of our earthly existence, he is speaking about in his consulting room and writing about here. In a world of conflicting expert opinion, of contradictory scientific surveys, of fads and fancies and fierce dietary debate, Warrick Bishop is leading us towards some diagnostic certainty. If we know what's actually happening inside, then we have a basis for remedial action.

In my case, Warrick Bishop tells me that if I lay off the carbs and keep the cholesterol down, I should get an extra couple of years in the Eventide Home. Maybe, eventually, I'll see you there. In the meantime, enjoy the book.

CHARLES WOOLEY

Hobart-based international television journalist and author

Hobart, Tasmania, Australia

上医医未病之病
中医医将病之病
下医医已病之病

～黄帝内经～

Superior doctors prevent the disease.
Mediocre doctors treat the disease before evident.
Inferior doctors treat the full-blown disease.

HAUG DEE: NAI-CHING

2600BC

first Chinese medical text

Introduction -
Not good enough!

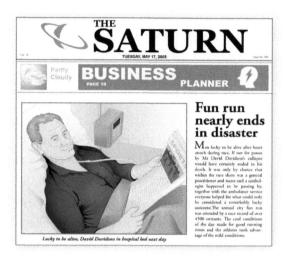

THE

SATURN

TUESDAY, MAY 17, 2005

Partly Cloudy

BUSINESS
PAGE 10 PLANNER

Fun run nearly ends in disaster

Man lucky to be alive after heart attack during race. If not for passes by Mr David Davidson's collapse would have certainly ended in his death. It was only by chance that within the race there was a general practitioner and nurse and a cardiologist happened to be passing by, together with the ambulance service everyone helped for what could only be considered a remarkably lucky outcome. The annual city fun run was attended by a race record of over 4500 entrants. The cool conditions of the day made for good running times and the athletes took advantage of the mild conditions.

Lucky to be alive, David Davidson in hospital bed next day

On a Saturday in May of 2005, a 52-year-old man collapsed, having had a cardiac arrest during a fun run. I noticed the commotion as I was driving past on my way to work and stopped. Several other runners, including a general practitioner, had already stopped to help and the Ambulance Service was in attendance. I am pleased to report that, with everyone's input, the man was resuscitated, taken to hospital and received stenting to the main artery down the front of his heart. The outcome was so good that it later made the front page of the local newspaper.

When I arrived at work on the Monday I felt fairly pleased to have been a contributor to such a positive outcome. Before I could become too proud, however, one of my staff pointed out that I had seen the very same gentleman two years earlier for an exercise treadmill test. The test had been normal and I had reassured him that "everything's okay". This revelation shocked me! Had I done the wrong thing by this man? Had I misinterpreted the test? Were there other factors of which I had not been aware? As it turned out, I had done nothing wrong; the test was appropriately reported and he was given reassurance consistent with his risk assessment at that time. In fact, I had suggested he start low-dose aspirin because of his history of mildly elevated blood pressure, for which he was on treatment.

Not good enough!

My original assessment in 2003 had limitations. This book is about how, with today's technology, we can do better – potentially much better. It is about improved dealing with risk through investigation and management. I do not wish, ever, to be in a situation again when I reassure a patient and then find that person has suffered a heart attack, let alone be involved in that person's resuscitation! That man's collapse was over 10 years ago and technology has changed so that we can deal with these situations in a different way.

According to the American Heart Association, about 790,000 Americans suffer a heart attack each year

According to the Heart Foundation, someone in the U.S. dies from heart disease about every 90 seconds.

'Heart attack' is a layman's term referring to a narrowing or blockage of the coronary arteries that can kill, or requires some form of medical intervention such as medication, time in a hospital, balloons or stents, or coronary artery bypass grafting.

As a cardiologist, I have not yet met a patient who expected to have a problem; patients do not put into their diaries "possible problem with my heart next week". **Yet, what if we could be forewarned about, or prepared for, a potential problem with our coronary arteries?**

What if we were able to put in place preventative measures that may avert a problem? What if we were able to take away the surprise of a heart attack occurring 'out of the blue' and replace possible fear with prepared understanding?

What if we could PLAN NOT to have a heart attack?

Primary prevention ...

PETER was a 35-year-old male with high cholesterol who had tried cholesterol-lowering tablets but had suffered aches and pains. He really didn't want to be on medication unless it was clearly indicated. At our first meeting, he was fit and well, and was not on any regular medication. There was no history of premature coronary artery disease in his family although both his parents had had elevated cholesterol. His lipid profile was:

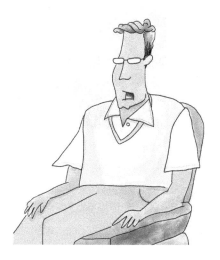

	mg/dl	mmol/l	ideally
Total Cholesterol (TC)	**450**	11.0	<(less than) **200/5.0**
Triglycerides (TG)	**75**	1.9	**<80/2.0**
High Density Lipoprotein (HDL)	**40**	1.0	>(greater than) **40/1.0**
TC to HDL ratio		11.0	<4.0 ratio
Non HDL	**385**	10.0	**<155/4.0**
Low Density Lipoprotein (LDL)	**350**	9.1	**<95/2.5**

These levels of cholesterol are high and concerning. The absolute cardiovascular disease risk calculator estimated Peter's risk at greater than 15 percent chance of an event in the next five years or over 30 percent in 10 years. This was a very high risk.

We spoke at some length about the role of scanning his heart to provide more information about the state of his arteries, in a bid to determine in more detail what his risk might be. I explained that he was younger than usual for such scanning. I also explained the risk of x-ray exposure and of possible contrast reactions.

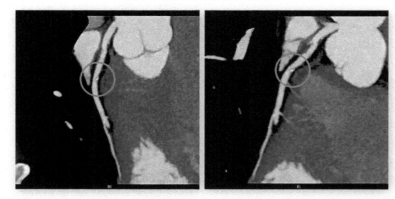

Peter was keen to undergo scanning so that he could be as well informed as possible and so make the best decisions for his care. He was married with three children and he didn't want to leave his heart health to chance. Above are the images we obtained.

The calcium score was three and this would generally suggest a low risk of an event over the next 5 to 10 years. However, as can be seen from the images above, there is a significant amount of non-calcific plaque which carries a high risk of an event over the next 5 to 10 years if left unattended.

I will explain plaque and other terminology soon.

This information was what Peter needed to know to be clear about his health management. I indicated that he would benefit from treatment. The pictures were explicit and gone were his doubts about the benefits of taking medication.

He is now on aspirin and two cholesterol-lowering medications, and has also embraced significant lifestyle changes. The result is a major turn-around in the management of his cardiovascular risk. He is happy with the outcome and is positive about being informed and proactive.

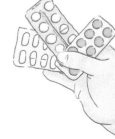

This is primary preventative cardiology – or much earlier intervention than traditionally undertaken – and is the fundamental focus of this book.

Treatment ...

Historically, the detection and the treatment of coronary artery disease have been related to either the presence of symptoms or the occurrence of an event, such as a heart attack. Once a patient has been diagnosed as having coronary heart disease, the way forward is very clear: re-establish or improve the blood flow and put in place secondary prevention strategies to reduce the risk of a recurrence. Methods used to reduce recurrence include use of medication, reducing cholesterol levels and lifestyle modifications.

The situation is not as clear-cut, however, when it involves patients who have not had a problem. They do not display any symptoms nor have they been defined as having a problem. Yet, they might be at high risk because of indicators such as cholesterol levels or high blood pressure or diabetes or even smoking.

The treatment for that risk, prior to an event, is *primary prevention* – and this is where our interest lies. The difficulty with primary prevention is that it involves **treatment of the unknown.**

Although important in its own right, secondary prevention of coronary artery disease, that treatment which happens after diagnosis, will not receive much attention in this book. The data around secondary prevention is very clear and I do not believe there is any need for an alternative interpretation. Its significance for me wearing my 'preventative cardiology' hat is, however, that secondary prevention is late, in fact potentially **too late,** in the process.

Let's avoid the first event ...

My objective in this book is to explore how to *avoid the first event*. When coronary artery disease is diagnosed at the time of the event, the time the patient has chest pain or shortness of breath or a major adverse coronary event, the patient has already developed a 'disease'. For me, to ***prevent*** chest pain or heart attack in the first place, to prevent the development of 'disease', is the Holy Grail of preventative cardiology.

Current primary prevention practice is based on *risk assessments*. I believe this has scope for re-evaluation.

The way we evaluate and calculate risk in individuals is based on **observational data.** This means that, over the years, databases have been compiled of features and factors found in individuals who have had coronary artery disease. The occurrence of those features and factors then lends weight to their being used as predictors for people before they have an event. Observational data collected from a large number of patients who have had heart attacks indicate that factors such as:

- increasing age;
- being male;
- cholesterol levels;
- increased blood pressure;
- diabetic status, and
- smoking

all feature as **associations** of having a possible a coronary event. The important thing is that these associations are not necessarily what has **caused** the problem. This means that there can be people who are high-risk based on such factors, yet they will not have an event.

Understanding that our risk evaluation is based on associations and not causations is central to the following discussion.

Another significant factor is that today's CT imaging of the heart offers us an ability to evaluate the health of an individual's arteries **before** the onset of a problem. **This is a paradigm shift in the conventional management of coronary artery disease.** Yet, although cardiac CT imaging has been generally available for the past five to 10 years, it has not yet been broadly taken up.

An exploration of the exciting opportunities that cardiac imaging offers is also crucial to this book.

Although formalised guidelines or recommendations do not exist for some of the issues I will cover, I plan to use a logical and systematic approach, based on science that is available today, to discuss the case for a much broader understanding and application of preventative cardiology. Based on this information, I extend a two-fold invitation:

- **to patients,** to engage their doctors in a meaningful discussion about their heart health and well-being, and

- **to doctors,** to look into these issues with an open mind, with the best patient outcome as a priority.

It is a win-win situation for everyone.

Let's explore ...

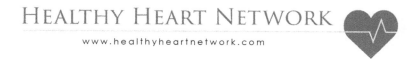

THE ULTIMATE MEMBERSHIP TO STAYING HEALTHY AND LIVING LONGER...

HEALTHY HEART NETWORK

www.healthyheartnetwork.com

The argument for a re-evaluation of our approach to primary prevention in cardiac health care management

As a GP, I have been referring patients to Dr Bishop for around 10 years now. When speaking with me later, patients who have seen Dr Bishop highlight his communication skills and say that he explains their cardiac conditions to them in such a way that they can easily understand and, therefore, they feel comfortable with their treatment. His approachable, down-to-earth manner makes patients feel respected and at ease.

Deborah Peters, GP, Hobart

Chapter 1 -
Understanding your heart

> the heart structure and its vulnerability

> symptoms and heart attack

No-one needs to be convinced about the importance of the heart for a healthy, well-functioning body. We all know that the heart is one of the critical organs necessary to sustain life.

The heart is a large muscle that pumps blood through our bodies to supply nutrients and oxygen, and also to remove waste such as carbon dioxide. It can be likened to a car engine, with compression chambers and valves, an electrical system and a set of fuel lines. Critical to the heart's operation are three major arteries, the coronary arteries. These are the fuel lines which carry blood to the heart muscle so that it can contract rhythmically, pumping blood to the body, 35 million times every year. As in a car engine, these lines can become blocked. This is the problem which concerns us.

CARDIOVASCULAR DISEASE involves heart and blood vessel diseases and includes stroke.

It affects over 92 million Americans, causing one death approximately every 40 seconds!

We all know people who have had heart problems and it is very likely that someone close to us, either family or friend, has suffered a heart attack or died after one. Although 'heart attack' is not a medical term, it is commonly used to refer to a major heart-related event that can end life or put the person in hospital. Such an event is most commonly associated with a full, or near-complete, occlusion, or blockage, of a coronary artery (one of the 'fuel lines') and the subsequent consequences.

Dealing with such events has focussed on the two-fold treatment of the consequences: firstly, understanding where the problem is so that improved blood flow can be re-established and secondly, trying to prevent recurrences. The way forward is clear: improve the blood flow and put in place preventative strategies to reduce the risk of any repeat events [1-3].

However, I believe there is another step which is often overlooked because the scientific evidence to support it is not as strong as for the above-mentioned best attempts to prevent the second heart attack. The issue around attempting to prevent problems **before** they manifest themselves with serious or fatal consequences is that the supporting data around the early detection of potential trouble is often anecdotal and not well supported by evidence-based trials and literature [4-7]. When trying to stave off repeat events, there are few such issues. A major cardiac event, an obvious problem, has occurred.

It is my contention that treatment can be instigated *before* clear indicators of a cardiac event are so obvious.

Typically, individual risk is evaluated using **associations** demonstrated in **population** studies. Yet, this presents inherent problems as the risk may be *low for the population* but it is *100 percent for the individual* who has the event!

***Symptoms* that point to *potential* problems in the coronary artery system are:**

- angina, or chest pain on exertion;
- shortness of breath on exertion, and
- acute coronary syndrome, manifested by chest pain at rest, leading to damage or death of part of the heart.

These are caused by:

- the build-up of plaque in the artery which
- leads to a narrowing of the vessel through which the blood is being pumped.

Plaque, **the build-up of cholesterol, scavenger cells, scar tissue and calcium in the wall of the artery which is generally very localised, can be linked to a variety of** *associations,* **including:**

- age;
- sex;
- smoking;
- cholesterol level;
- high blood pressure, and/or
- diabetes

Which can combine to influence the development of coronary artery disease.

This early, or **primary,** prevention which I am advocating attempts to prevent the development of coronary disease in a patient who has not suffered an event but indicators suggest could be at risk.

Before discussing more precise evaluation for primary prevention, we need to look at some basics.

Groundwork: the heart

Let's return to the analogy of our car engine.

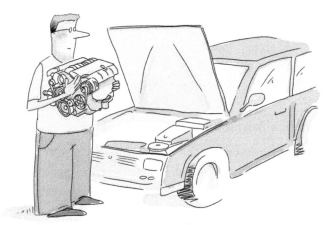

As a car engine has an **electrical system** for timing, so does the heart. The electrical system in the heart ensures synchronicity and coordinated contraction throughout the heart. It also allows a mechanism for acceleration and deceleration.

A car has **pistons** and **valves.** This is the engine block, the part that generates the power. So, within the heart, the pistons are the compression chambers, the main one being the **ventricle,** and the valves which stop the blood flowing back from where it came.

The car engine also requires a **fuel line** to supply the engine block. In the human heart, the fuel lines are the **coronary arteries** that literally provide the life blood to the engine block, the muscle that is the heart.

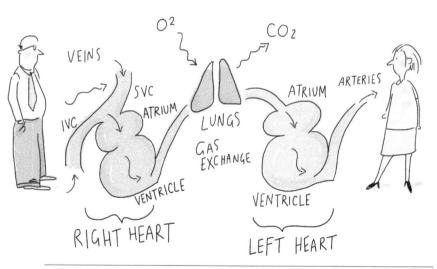

A schematic showing the flow of the blood through the heart from the veins to the arteries.

The heart is a four-chambered structure.

There are two chambers on the right-hand side and two chambers on the left-hand side. On each side of the heart there is a pre-pumping chamber, the **atrium,** and a main pumping chamber, the **ventricle.** There is a right-sided and a left-sided ventricle. The muscle of the heart is called the **myocardium** (*myo* meaning muscle and *cardium,* being of the heart).

Blood drains from the body through the veins, collecting into two major veins called the **superior vena cava** (SVC) and the **inferior vena cava** (IVC) which drain into the right side of the heart. This blood arrives in the right atrium and is given a gentle pump through a one-way valve into the ventricle which then pumps the blood through another one-way valve into the lungs. Within the lungs, gas exchange occurs: oxygen is absorbed from the air we breathe in and carbon dioxide is released through the breath we exhale.

The blood then flows from the lungs to the left atrium. The left atrium gives a gentle pump and the blood passes through the mitral valve, a one-way valve, into the left ventricle which then contracts, squeezing blood through the aortic valve into the main artery of the body, the **aorta,** as it begins its journey around the body. The contraction of the left ventricle makes the blood flow through the arteries that we can feel pulsating under the skin.

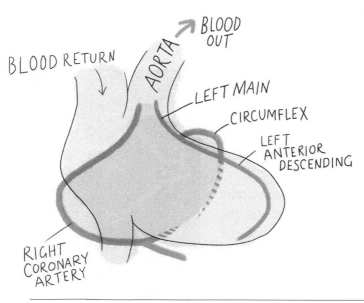

A schematic showing how the blood vessels wrap around the heart.

The coronary arteries arise from the aorta as it comes from the left ventricle. They are the first branches in the circulation.

It is useful to think of the arteries as the fuel lines supplying the cylinders of the car, transporting blood to different territories (pistons) of the heart muscle. This system consists of the **right coronary artery** and **left main coronary artery.** Within one centimetre, the left coronary artery divides into two main arteries: the **left anterior descending artery** which provides blood to the anterior surface of the heart, that is the surface nearest the chest wall, and the **circumflex artery** which supplies blood to the back of the heart or the surface of the heart nearest the spine. The **right coronary artery** supplies the inferior surface of the heart or the surface that is nearest the diaphragm.

The terms 'right dominant' or 'left dominant' can be used in reference to the origin of the artery that supplies blood to the bulk of the inferior surface of the heart. This is generally from the right coronary artery but sometimes the right coronary is smaller and the circumflex is 'dominant', or bigger, supplying the majority of the inferior surface of the heart. This is called 'left dominant'. This becomes important in terms of the amount of the heart that may be affected by a blockage of the artery, the dominant artery providing blood to a larger territory.

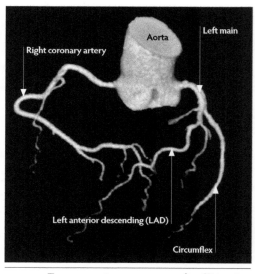

The left anterior descending artery supplies blood to the anterior wall of the heart (nearest the chest wall). Most often, the left anterior descending artery is the largest and most important of the three main coronary arteries.

The coronary tree as seen on cardiac CT imaging.

It can be 12cm to 14cm long, while only two to five millimetres in diameter. This is little thicker than a pen refill, yet its blockage can be disastrous. A dominant right coronary artery can be approximately the same size and a non-dominant circumflex can be six to eight centimetres long and 1.5 to three millimetres in diameter.

The major arteries comprise fewer than 35cm in total length and fewer than five millimetres in diameter at their largest. A single build-up of plaque leading to a blockage may only be one centimetre in length. **This is not a system with a lot of redundancy, making it very vulnerable.**

Groundwork: the blood

The heart pumps three to four litres of blood every minute.

It is important to be aware of the contents of the blood.

The blood contains **red cells** which are carriers of **haemoglobin,** the oxygen-carrying substance which transports oxygen to the body's tissues. It is critical for the metabolism of the heart, or the normal working of the heart muscle, to receive a good supply of oxygen.

The other important components of the blood are the **platelets.** These small particles are central in forming clots or *thrombi* when damage is detected within the vascular system. Platelets stop the bleeding, for example, when we cut ourselves.

The blood also carries **nutrients** and fats such as **cholesterol.**

Coronary artery disease

Historically, it has not been possible to medically evaluate the coronary arteries in a well person. So, the first time that a problem with the arteries can be suspected is when symptoms (angina, shortness of breath or an acute coronary syndrome) present.

Angina is the term given to discomfort in the chest when pain is experienced in association with exertion. The term has its root meaning in a sense of strangulation.

Shortness of breath on exertion can indicate a lack of blood flowing to the heart. Under these circumstances the heart cannot work properly, pressures within the pumping chamber begin to rise with back pressure to the lungs and, consequently, the person experiences shortness of breath.

An **acute coronary syndrome** is the sudden development of a complete, or near complete, occlusion, or blockage, of a coronary artery. A lessened blood flow to a region of heart muscle results in damage. A complete blockage causes the death of that area of the heart muscle. This is called a **myocardial infarction** (*myo,* muscle, *cardiam,* heart; *infarction,* death by lack of blood flow). A near complete blockage, or 'unstable angina', puts strain on the heart and can be a forerunner to a complete blockage, or heart attack.

About 635,000 people in the U.S. have a first-time heart attack each year, and about 300,000 have recurrent heart attacks.

The medical term for 'heart attack', a full blockage or near-complete blockage of a coronary artery and its consequences, is **Major Adverse Coronary Event** or **MACE.** *(Heart attack is used in this book in the context of a major adverse coronary event and the terms will be used interchangeably.)*

Another important term in this discussion is **plaque.** This is the build-up of cholesterol, scavenger cells, scar tissue and calcium in the wall of the artery. The medical terminology for the build-up of these materials is **atherosclerotic plaque.** For simplicity, we will call this 'plaque' and at times simplify the process to a 'build-up of cholesterol in the arteries'. Plaque is localised. It occurs where wear and tear of the artery have led it to develop.

The term ***coronary artery disease* describes the process of atherosclerosis or plaque build-up in the arteries that leads to impaired blood flow which causes symptoms or loss of function.**

We know from observation that coronary artery disease is a patchy process. Autopsies on patients who have died from coronary artery disease have shown that generally a focal, localised area or lesion, or plaque has led to the life-ending event. Within the same artery, there can be areas that may not be diseased to the same extent, or even at all.

This is particularly significant when we consider sudden cardiac death. Most people can deal conceptually with the idea of some shortness of breath or chest pain on exertion. My own grandfather, for example, for a number of years had angina when he walked too far up the street or rushed while undertaking his daily activities. The real issue that concerns most of us is sudden cardiac death.

Could I please emphasise to the reader that these symptoms need to be taken seriously.

PLEASE, PLEASE, PLEASE seek immediate medical attention should you be affected by chest pain or unexplained shortness of breath.

Autopsies after sudden cardiac death from coronary artery disease show that about 60 percent of the culprit lesions or plaques have been **flow-limiting,** or tight, prior to the event that led to death and, hence, likely to have given a clue by way of a symptom such as chest pain or shortness of breath.

This leaves about 40 percent that has been **non-flow-limiting** before the event. In this situation, the person has no warning at all and so no chance to seek help before the event. This is the group in which death strikes suddenly and without warning, often in a seemingly fit and healthy person. **This is critical to our understanding of how we might be able to prevent death from coronary artery disease.**

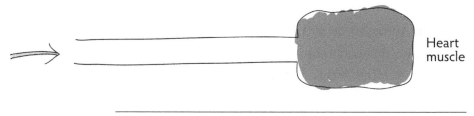

A schematic of a blood vessel supplying heart muscle.

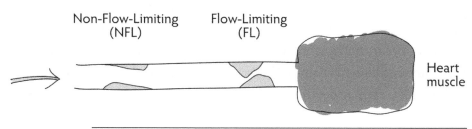

A schematic showing build up of non-flow-limiting and flow-limiting plaque in the artery.

If we were to cut through the plaque (either the flow-limiting or non-flow-limiting) we would see similar components:

- the wall of the artery;
- the lumen (or inside space) of the artery;
- the cholesterol plaque which has built up and is beginning to intrude into the artery, and
- a fibrous cap that separates the plaque from the blood.

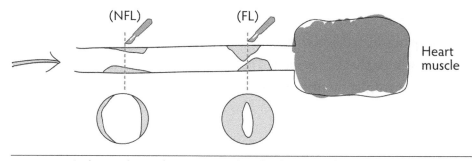

A schematic showing the components of non-flow-limiting and flow-limiting plaque are the same, just to a different extent.

The blood contains many different components. Importantly, there are platelets, those small particles responsible for the formation of a clot when any abnormality is detected in the inside lining of the artery. In an **unstable plaque,** rupture of the fibrous cap covering the build-up of cholesterol can occur. The blood comes into contact with the content of the plaque. The platelets, having rapidly detected the change, start to clump together to form a clot which may progress to a complete blockage of the artery.

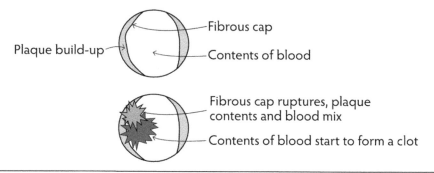

A schematic showing how, when the contents of the plaque come into contact with the contents of the blood, the body begins to form a clot.

This is so concerning because a non-flow-limiting plaque will give absolutely no symptoms, no clues, no warning. Even a microscopic tear in the fibrous cap of a plaque can lead to the formation of a clot, which can then rapidly block off that artery and be life-ending.

Ten to 15 percent of people who suffer a heart attack die[8,9], and many will have no prior warning.

AN INTERESTING POINT: If we were to suffer a cut, the platelets would clump at the site of the wound and save us from bleeding to death. In the setting of a ruptured plaque, the very thing platelets are meant to do can cause death.

IMPORTANT POINTS

- Detection and treatment of coronary artery disease, historically, has been related to the presence of symptoms or the occurrence of a major coronary event.

- Plaque is related to the build-up of cholesterol and other matter within the arteries. This build-up can be patchy, tending to occur where there are points of stress, weakness and/or vulnerability in the artery.

- Plaque can be flow-limiting (which generally, though not always, produces symptoms) or non-flow-limiting (which will cause no symptoms). However, in either case, unstable plaque can rupture and a clot, which can block the artery, can form very quickly. When a seemly fit and healthy person drops dead, during exercise, for example, it is often the case that the person had an unstable non-flow- limiting plaque rupture (and therefore, no symptoms before the life-ending event).

[1]   Abed MA, Khalil AA, Moser DK. Awareness of modifiable acute myocardial infarction risk factors has little impact on risk perception for heart attack among vulnerable patients. Heart Lung 2015;44:183-8.

[2]   Hoevenaar-Blom MP, Spijkerman AM, Boshuizen HC, Boer JM, Kromhout D, Verschuren WM. Effect of using repeated measurements of a Mediterranean style diet on the strength of the association with cardiovascular disease during 12 years: the Doetinchem Cohort Study. Eur J Nutr 2014;53:1209-15.

[3]   Lanas F, Avezum A, Bautista LE, et al. Risk factors for acute myocardial infarction in Latin America: the INTERHEART Latin American study. Circulation 2007;115:1067-74.

[4]   Celermajer DS, Chow CK, Marijon E, Anstey NM, Woo KS. Cardiovascular disease in the developing world: prevalences, patterns, and the potential of early disease detection. J Am Coll Cardiol 2012;60:1207-16.

[5]   Scandinavian Simvastatin Survival Study G. Randomised trial of cholesterol lowering in 4444 patients with coronary heart disease: the Scandinavian Simvastatin Survival Study (4S). The Lancet 1994;344:1383-89.

[6]   Ford I, Murray H, Packard CJ, Shepherd J, Macfarlane PW, Cobbe SM. Long-
       Term Follow-up of the West of Scotland Coronary Prevention Study. New England
       Journal of Medicine 2007;357:1477-86.

[7]   Sutton L, Karan A, Mahal A. Evidence for cost-effectiveness of lifestyle primary
       preventions for cardiovascular disease in the Asia-Pacific Region: a systematic
       review. Globalization and Health 2014;10:1-19.

[8]   Libby P, Ridker PM, Hansson GK. Progress and challenges in translating the
       biology of atherosclerosis. Nature 2011;473:317-25.

[9]   Aso S, Imamura H, Sekiguchi Y, et al. Incidence and mortality of acute myocardial
       infarction. A population-based study including patients with out-of-hospital
       cardiac arrest. Int Heart J 2011;52:197-202.

Now that we have a basic understanding of the heart, the next chapter looks at the current approach to discovering and treating coronary artery disease.

Chapter 2 -
A current approach

IN THIS CHAPTER WE LOOK AT

> primary and secondary prevention

> population risk vs individual risk

> risk, association and causation

> understanding screening

Our approach to coronary artery disease tends mainly to focus on secondary prevention or dealing with the consequences of the disease: the symptoms and signs associated with a shortage of blood flowing to the heart, including shortness of breath, chest pain on exertion or an acute coronary syndrome.

On having diagnosed a patient, treatment is based on:

- understanding exactly where the problems are within the coronary arteries so that decisions can be made about whether re-establishing or improving blood flow with the use of technology such as stents or coronary artery bypass grafting is appropriate – **revascularisation,** and

- trying to prevent another event or a further problem occurring – **secondary prevention.**

Strategies to reduce the risk of a recurrence, include:

- » the **use of medication**[1] to keep the platelets from clumping together and forming blockages in the arteries; aspirin is most commonly used for this;

- » **reducing cholesterol levels**[1] to known targets associated with a significant improvement in outcome, often using cholesterol-lowering agents such as statins, and

» **life-style modifications**[2] that may reduce the risk, including exercise, weight loss, treatment of high blood pressure and/or diabetes, stopping smoking.

There is no question that secondary prevention is beneficial in reducing the recurrence of an event[3]. These patients clearly have a significant build-up of cholesterol in their arteries. The data around secondary prevention is very clear and I do not believe there is any need for alternative interpretations or strategies.

While my patients would tell you I adopt an almost boot camp mentality in my use of secondary prevention measures, from my perspective, the timing of secondary prevention is late in the process. You wouldn't want to die on your way to secondary prevention!

The problem is that the situation is not so sharply defined when it involves patients who have not yet had a problem. They may be at high-risk because of indicators such as cholesterol levels or blood pressure, or diabetes, or even smoking, yet they do not display any symptoms, nor have they been defined as having a problem. Even so, these patients may carry an increased risk. The treatment for that risk, **prior** to an event, is **primary prevention.**

My objective is to explore ways to avoid the first event. I believe that current primary prevention practice has scope for a *re-evaluation of our approach to risk assessment in individuals* before they even have a problem. For me, to prevent the chest pain or the heart attack in the first place is the Holy Grail of preventative cardiology.

The difficulty with primary prevention is that it involves the unrevealed:

- consideration of treatment before there is a clear indication as to whether or not an individual has a significant build-up of plaque within the arteries;
- whether or not the person has genuine high-risk features, and
- the probability of an event.

Defining risk

Within cardiology terminology, we define the risk of a coronary artery event as "low", "intermediate" or "high". A **low** risk is considered a less than 10 percent chance of a coronary event within 10 years. A **high** risk is considered a greater than 20 percent chance of an event within 10 years. An **intermediate** risk is between 10 and 20 percent risk of an event within 10 years.

This means that, if we were to take a group of 100 people who were high-risk and follow them for 10 years, 20 or more of those people would have a coronary event or symptom. If we introduced aspirin and a cholesterol-lowering tablet to reduce the risk of an event in this group of 100 then, statistically, we would be treating up to 80 people who were not going to have an event and perhaps did not need treatment. This has a significant impact on the way the effectiveness of that intervention is assessed. The statistical significance of assessing the effectiveness of primary prevention in this group is diluted by the people within the population who were not destined to have an event.

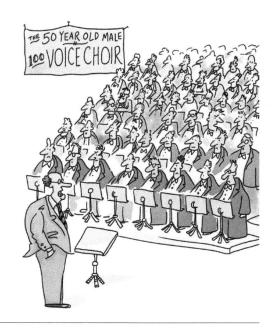

Similarly, if we were to take a group of 100 people with low risk of an event and follow them for 10 years, up to 10 of those individuals could have a coronary event and 90 would remain without any symptom or sign. Here again, the problem is: *How do we appropriately treat the 10 but not over-treat the 90?*

"OK guys, I've spoken to the doc and he says 10 to 15 of you will have a heart attack in the next 10 years. Could I just ask that it's not all the tenors?"

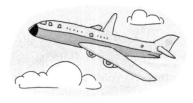

Interestingly, within the context of our medical classification, we are happy to refer to low risk as up to a 10 percent chance within 10 years and not consider treatment, even though this could be expressed as a one percent chance per annum of having a major event. How would you react if, the next time you booked a commercial airline flight, you were told there was a one percent per annum chance of being involved in a crash, or a 10 percent chance of being involved in a crash over your next 10 years of flying?

The way that we evaluate and calculate risk in individuals is based on **observational** data. This means that, over years, databases have been collated of features and factors found in individuals who have had coronary artery disease. The occurrence of those features and factors then lends weight to their being used as **predictors** for people **before they have an event.** This simply means that observational data collected on a large number of patients who have had heart attacks indicate that factors such as increasing age, being male, increased blood pressure, diabetic status and smoking all feature as **associations** to having had a coronary event.

This type of risk modelling, using multiple associations with observed outcomes, was first widely published and used by the **Framingham** Group[4]. This Framingham-type risk modelling continues to form the basis of our current risk assessment in primary prevention[5].

The interesting thing about this, of course, is that these factors are **associations,** and not necessarily **causations,** the mechanisms that actually cause the problem. This means that there can be people who are high-risk based on factors such as age, sex and cholesterol levels, yet never have an event. Conversely, there are people who would appear to score low on these risk calculators but still manage to have a coronary problem.

Understanding that our current risk evaluation is based on associations, and that those associations do not always necessarily have a direct link to the causation of the development of plaque within the arteries, is central to the discussion I wish to have throughout the remainder of this book.

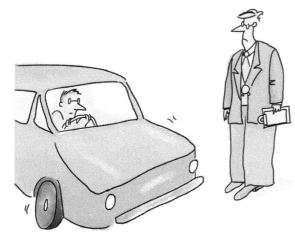

Let's look at this from outside the medical field. We know that speeding and alcohol consumption are significant associations of car accidents. However, we also know that people do drive over the speed limit with high alcohol levels, yet do not have an accident. Conversely, we know that people who drive safely can be involved in an accident. This does not mean that driving within the speed limit and not consuming alcohol when driving are wastes of time. **It simply alters the risk profile.** It means that speed and alcohol are **associations** with having an accident. If they were **causations,** then every time someone sped or had consumed alcohol, that person would crash.

When it comes to the heart, being aware of your blood pressure and keeping it down, being aware of your cholesterol

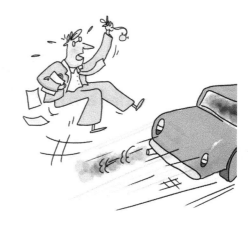

and dealing with it appropriately, undertaking regular exercise, not smoking and addressing other cardiovascular risks are all important for a safe journey through life. However, **on their own,** they offer **no guarantee** of avoiding a heart attack, although they are likely to **reduce the risk.** Remember the fun runner in the introduction: he was active, exercised regularly and had appropriate treatment for his blood pressure, yet that didn't protect him.

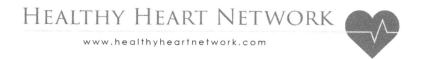

THE ULTIMATE MEMBERSHIP TO STAYING HEALTHY AND LIVING LONGER...

HEALTHY HEART NETWORK

www.healthyheartnetwork.com

association vs causation

In discussing issues around **risk factor assessment** in relation to coronary artery disease, it is extremely important to be clear about the difference between **association** and **causation.**

Regularly, I need to advise patients that they have cholesterol build-up in their arteries.

Invariably I receive the reply,

- "But Doctor, my cholesterol is fine."
- "But Doctor, I exercise regularly."
- "But Doctor, I eat healthy food and keep my weight down."

These patients are expressing a belief which is **broadly accepted** but **universally misleading:** that certain factors, such as elevated cholesterol, lack of exercise, eating poorly or being overweight are the **direct causes** of coronary artery disease.

They are not the *causes*; they are *associations*.

If we were to return to our alcohol and driving example: alcohol is associated with an increased incidence of car accidents. Alcohol does not cause the car accident; it does not drive the car, yet alcohol can impair the driver's reflexes and assessment and **contribute** to that driver having an accident.

The actual **cause** of the accident may be approaching a sharp bend too quickly, a car in front stopping unexpectedly, changing the radio and losing concentration, or a dog running out on to the street.

In fact, a car accident is an excellent example when trying to understand association and causation. Multiple associations can be present such as alcohol, speeding, driver inexperience, poor weather. These associations, even when put together, do not necessarily mean that that car will be involved in an accident, just that there is **a higher risk.**

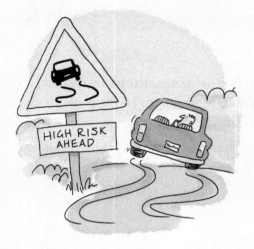

The reverse is true also. There may be no alcohol, no speeding, an experienced driver in good weather and yet, without any associations present, an accident occurs.

Our lack of understanding of the exact mechanisms of the development of coronary artery disease in a single individual, in a particular artery, at a particular location within the artery, means that our science around coronary artery disease is based on the science of **observation,** not the science of **mechanism.** Consequently, that science of observation leads to a clearer understanding of **association.**

The reason for highlighting this is that **there is a substantial gap between association and causation, and it is this gap that I hope to shed light on in subsequent chapters.**

We know, both from literature and from personal experience, of people with high cholesterol levels who do not have heart attacks, of people who exercise regularly and have a heart attack, seemingly out of the blue at a young age, of people who smoke, are overweight and do not exercise who live long lives without problems, and we see family clusters in which major adverse coronary events occur at a much higher frequency but not in all members.

Problems for primary prevention

Currently, the data that supports primary prevention is pretty thin[6-8].

Certainly in some **high**-risk groups, such as patients who have familial hypercholesterolaemia, there is no question that studies have shown primary prevention is beneficial. Hypercholesterolaemia is a genetic condition which gives rise to very elevated levels of cholesterol and is associated with a family history of premature coronary artery disease[9]. There is also reasonable data to support that high-risk patients, if appropriately selected, will benefit from intervention such as aspirin, lowered cholesterol, treatment of diabetes and lowered blood pressure, targeted in a primary prevention role[3,9].

The Achilles Heel of primary prevention arises in the **intermediate**-risk and **low**-risk populations. These groups, with the majority of the population being unlikely to have a problem, will need to be treated, accepting that they may not have an event over the next 10 or even 20 year period. Statistically, the effectiveness of a primary prevention regime, therefore, is markedly diluted and the cost of drugs, and side-effects associated with drugs, are spread across a large number of people who probably do not need them. The unfortunate consequence of this is that the 10 to 15 percent of people, who may appear to be at low to intermediate risk but will have an event and who may benefit, do not represent enough numbers to make these studies appear worthwhile or this intervention effective.

I will discuss in later chapters ways that we could become more precise around evaluating risk in the individual and therefore being more targeted in our approach to risk modification. This in turn, I believe, would make the process more efficient and more cost effective, and would improve the risk/benefit profile of the medications involved.

Screening using stress tests

Before moving on to that detail, however, I would like to mention a part of our current approach that I believe has some **significant limitations: stress testing as an indicator of coronary artery disease.** The exercise stress test, usually undertaken on a treadmill or a stationary exercise bike, is used to determine how blood is flowing through the arteries.

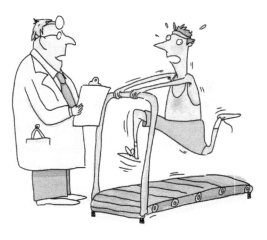

Health insurance companies and other agencies and organisations still use stress testing as an indicator of coronary artery disease. For example, there are guidelines within the Civil Aviation Safety Authority which dictate that pilots, beyond a certain age, should have regular stress testing. Until recently, this was a fair and reasonable thing to do, as it was, in fact, the only way we could try to unmask a problem within the arteries in a non-invasive and objective fashion. Available data suggest that if a patient performs well on a treadmill test without evidence of any problems, then his/her one year mortality, or risk of a major problem, is low[10]. Remember it was 'low' for the fun runner in the introduction.

By recalling our earlier discussion, you will appreciate that there is a limitation to this testing: that a significant amount of **cholesterol** or **atheroma** can build in the arteries **before** it actually leads to a narrowing and, therefore, before it shows any features on stress testing. Thus, it is fairly late in the process when it shows up. To a degree, that patient has run the gauntlet of a major event with potential rupture of the non-flow-limiting plaque which would remain undetectable because it causes no limitation to flow until the moment it ruptures.

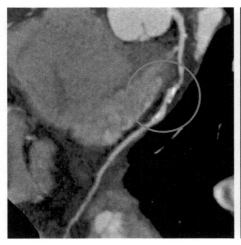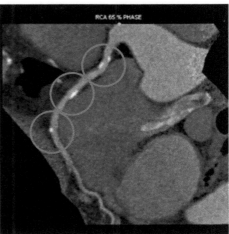

These are images from a cardiac CT scan done on a 61-year-old fireman who had had a "normal" exercise stress test, exercising for 12 minutes without problems. He still wanted more reassurance as he had a history of high blood pressure, and there was a family history of coronary disease and diabetes.

The scans clearly show a significant build-up of plaque that could not be picked up by the stress testing. This additional information allowed for appropriate risk management that otherwise would not have been undertaken.

I believe and hope some of the discussion that follows may reframe the approach to cardiovascular health assessment in situations for pilots, commercial drivers, emergency workers and the armed forces, and in insurance evaluations, as well as for the general population.

IMPORTANT POINTS

- Primary prevention aims at stopping someone from having a heart attack or developing heart problems. Scientific evidence to support this is not as strong as for secondary prevention, or preventing a second heart attack or recurrence of a problem.

- In evaluating for risk of an individual in primary prevention, we use associations which have been demonstrated in population studies. This presents an inherent problem as risk may be low for the population but is 100 percent for the individual who has an event.

- Individual screening using stress testing, as employed in some organisational settings, will pick up problems only late in the process of cholesterol build-up in the arteries.

[1] Fleg JL, Forman DE, Berra K, et al. Secondary Prevention of Atherosclerotic Cardiovascular Disease in Older Adults: A Scientific Statement From the American Heart Association. Circulation 2013;128:2422-46.

[2] Eckel RH, Jakicic JM, Ard JD, et al. 2013 AHA/ACC Guideline on Lifestyle Management to Reduce Cardiovascular Risk: A Report of the American College of Cardiology/American Heart Association Task Force on Practice Guidelines. Circulation 2014;129:S76-S99.

[3] Abed MA, Khalil AA, Moser DK. Awareness of modifiable acute myocardial infarction risk factors has little impact on risk perception for heart attack among vulnerable patients. Heart Lung 2015;44:183-8.

[4] Kannel WB, McGee D, Gordon T. A general cardiovascular risk profile: The Framingham study. The American Journal of Cardiology 1976;38:46-51.

[5] Greenland P, LaBree L, Azen SP, Doherty TM, Detrano RC. Coronary artery calcium score combined with Framingham score for risk prediction in asymptomatic individuals. Jama 2004;291:210-5.

[6] Sutton L, Karan A, Mahal A. Evidence for cost-effectiveness of lifestyle primary preventions for cardiovascular disease in the Asia-Pacific Region: a systematic review. Globalization and Health 2014;10:1-19.

[7]   *Scandinavian Simvastatin Survival Study G. Randomised trial of cholesterol lowering in 4444 patients with coronary heart disease: the Scandinavian Simvastatin Survival Study (4S). The Lancet 1994;344:1383-89.*

[8]   *Ford I, Murray H, Packard CJ, Shepherd J, Macfarlane PW, Cobbe SM. Long-Term Follow-up of the West of Scotland Coronary Prevention Study. New England Journal of Medicine 2007;357:1477-86.*

[9]   *Watts GF, Sullivan DR, Poplawski N, et al. Familial hypercholesterolaemia: a model of care for Australasia. Atheroscler Suppl 2011;12:221-63.*

[10]   *Shaw LJ, Peterson ED, Shaw LK, et al. Use of a prognostic treadmill score in identifying diagnostic coronary disease subgroups. Circulation 1998;98:1622-30.*

The next chapter presents several case studies to help further set the scene.

Chapter 3 -
A picture paints a thousand words

> several very different case studies

One of the key tools to my approach to primary prevention is to use the latest technology available to scan the heart. We will go into detail in later chapters but for the moment it is enough to appreciate that, by scanning the heart, I can obtain as much information as possible about the condition of the arteries of the patient's heart by looking at the arteries literally to see what is going on.

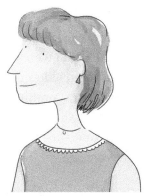

As 'a picture paints a thousand words', here are some 'patient pictures' as examples.

KAREN was a 60-year-old woman who came to see me for cardiovascular risk stratification. She was generally fit and well, not on any regular medication and there was no history of premature coronary artery disease in her family. Her cholesterol profile was:

	mg/dl	mmol/l	ideally
Total Cholesterol (TC)	**350**	9.1	< (less than) **200/5.0**
Triglycerides (TG)	**80**	2.0	<**80/2.0**
High Density Lipoprotein (HDL)	**80**	2.1	> (greater than)**40/1.0**
TC to HDL ratio		4.3	<4.0 ratio
Non HDL	**280**	7.0	<**155/4.0**
Low Density Lipoprotein (LDL)	**240**	6.1	<**95**2.5

This was her cardiovascular disease risk factor calculator result.

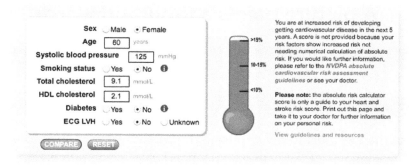

This was not a good result. The calculator estimated her risk at greater than a 15 percent chance of an event in the next five years, or over 30 percent in 10 years. This was a very high risk, so high that she had a red thermometer!

It transpired that, over the years, each time Karen had visited her doctor, she had been given a script for a cholesterol-lowering tablet; each time she had suffered side-effects and had stopped taking the tablets within weeks. We spoke at length about using CT to image the heart, to provide more detail regarding the 'health' of her arteries. Karen agreed as she was eager to see what was really going on.

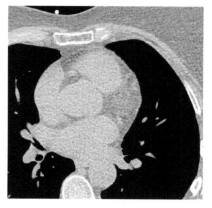

This is the scan result for Karen. Her coronary calcium score was zero. There was no evidence of plaque build-up at all, despite her cholesterol levels. We did not undertake further evaluation.

This result was a fantastic relief to Karen who had been stressed by the desire of her local doctor to have her on a cholesterol-lowering tablet, not withstanding the side-effects she suffered. She was caught between the fear of an event and the side-effects of medication.

Based on the above scan, I could reassure her that all the available research suggests that the presence of a zero calcium score was a very low-risk feature, likely to represent a risk of event of less than one percent in 10 years (all things being equal). We discussed this at some length and agreed on a plan of management. As there was no evidence of plaque, there appeared to be no benefit for her in taking a statin or aspirin. However, we acknowledged that the literature's suggestion of a very low risk of an event over 10 years might not be the situation in her case because of the higher than average cholesterol level. So to err on the side of caution, we decided to repeat the scan in five years and reconsider treatment based on that next result.

A demonstrated low risk of event informed the immediate medication decision, which was backed up by a plan for ongoing surveillance. Karen was happy with the outcome.

....

TWO SISTERS, TRACEY and BECK, came to see me. Both had elevated cholesterol levels and there was a family history of premature coronary artery disease. They were in their early 50s and neither wanted to take cholesterol-lowering medication unless it were really necessary. Their cholesterol profiles were: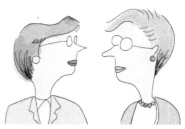

Tracey:

	mg/dl	mmol/l	ideally
Total Cholesterol (TC)	315	8.2	< (less than) **200/5.0**
Triglycerides (TG)	85	2.2	<**80/2.0**
High Density Lipoprotein (HDL)	40	1.0	> (greater than) **40/1.0**
TC to HDL ratio		8.2	<4.0 ratio
Non HDL	280	7.2	<**155/4.0**
Low Density Lipoprotein (LDL)	240	6.2	<**95/2.5**

Beck:

	mg/dl	mmol/l	ideally
Total Cholesterol (TC)	**420**	10.6	< (less than) **200/5.0**
Triglycerides (TG)	**465**	12.5	**<80/2.0**
High Density Lipoprotein (HDL)	**30**	0.8	> (greater than) **40/1.0**
TC to HDL ratio		13.3	<4.0 ratio
Non HDL	**380**	9.8	**<155/4.0**

(LDL) unable to be measured accurately because of high TG

For both sisters, the cardiovascular disease risk calculator suggested a risk of an event of greater than 15 percent in five years. After discussing the pros and cons of using cardiac CT, both sisters proceeded with the testing.

These are the results:

Tracey

This is a zero calcium score and suggests a low risk of coronary event in the next 5 to 10 years.

Tracey's scan for coronary calcium score

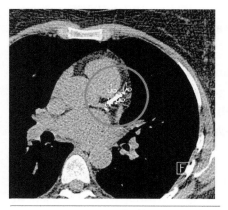

Beck's coronary calcuim

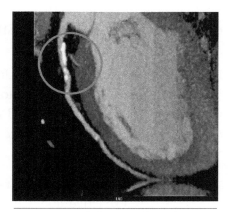

Left anterior descending artery

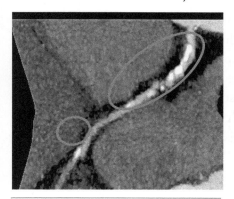

Right coronary artery

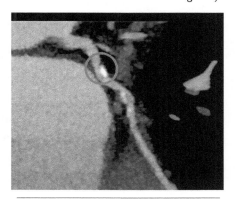

Circumflex artery

Beck

For Beck, the calcium score was over 1000. This was very high and, in comparison with 100 women of the same age taken randomly from the population, would be at least in the highest five (above the 95th percentile), perhaps even the highest.

Even without experience at looking at cardiac CT images, it can be seen that the pictures clearly show a significant build-up of plaque in all three arteries.

Beck's scans suggest very **high-risk** features.

These may be two sisters with the same family history and both with elevated cholesterol. However, the health of their arteries couldn't be more different. And no, I can't explain it.

Nonetheless, the information was clear and allowed a management strategy based on **exactly** what was seen to be going on in the arteries, not a best guess based on a population-based **probability** of what may be going on. *(The importance of this will become much clearer in subsequent chapters.)*

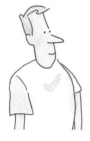

TONY was 63 years old when he came to see me. He was proactive about his health and wanted to be as clear as possible about his cardiac risk. When I saw him, he was taking a cholesterol-lowering tablet although it was a low dose and not aimed at the targets for a high-risk patient. He was not on aspirin. Interestingly, at his own initiation, he had undergone two treadmill stress tests (through another centre) in the previous two years and had been reassured everything was fine. When he came to see me he just wanted as much information as possible to be clear he was addressing his cardiovascular risk appropriately. This was his lipid profile:

	mg/dl	mmol/l	ideally
Total Cholesterol (TC)	140	3.6	< (less than) **200**/ 5.0
Triglycerides (TG)	55	1.4	< **80**/ 2.0
High Density Lipoprotein (HDL)	25	0.7	> (greater than) **40**/ 1.0
TC to HDL ratio		5.1	<4.0 ratio
Non HDL	110	2.9	<**55**/ 4.0
Low Density Lipoprotein (LDL)	85	2.2	< **95**/ 2.5

These numbers look pretty good, so why worry? Well, we spoke at length and Tony was eager to proceed to imaging of his heart arteries for his own peace of mind.

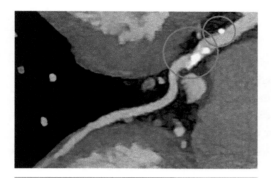

Tony's right coronary artery

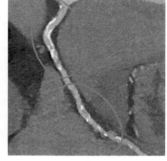

His circumflex artery

As you can see he has significant build-up. In fact, his calcium score was so high, it fell above the 90th percentile for his age group. The features were of very high risk for a coronary event.

With this information, we have, of course, commenced aspirin; we have increased his lipid-lowering therapy and improved his lipid profile in keeping with current guidelines. It has also been valuable in providing a focus to maximise lifestyle changes. The other important factor is that Tony is now well educated. Should there be **any** symptom that could be related to his heart, he knows to present for medical attention immediately. This education on its own could be life saving.

Tony was very pleased to have gone through the testing and to be better informed. There is no question that we have been able to improve his therapy in relation to his actual risk based on the state of his arteries. He realised that the stress tests had told him that he was 'fit' but had not told him the 'fitness' of his arteries.

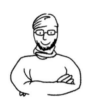 *I found it interesting that Tony had been given a statin for cardiovascular risk but had not been given aspirin. Debate surrounds the role of the broad use of aspirin for reducing risk in primary prevention[1]. The current recommendation is that it is not indicated. This is also the case in diabetes[2]. Tony's situation seemed odd; either he had an increased risk of heart attack or stroke and deserved treatment, or not. To use one but not the other seems to me like not using the seat belt because your car has an airbag. Why wouldn't you use all the safety features?*

Data suggest that aspirin is beneficial for a patient who is having a heart attack or who has had a heart attack[3,4]. So why wouldn't you give it to patients who seem to be at high risk of an event?

The answer is because there is no evidence it is beneficial if given to patients before an event. It seems logical to me that if you could give aspirin to the patient who is about to have a heart attack, it should help that person in the same way as a patient who has had a heart attack.

Later, I will discuss how we can better identify those high-risk patients by scanning their hearts, a technique not used in the studies looking at the role of aspirin in primary prevention. I will also talk about how the evidence base that we use in medicine to help decision-making and to formulate guidelines may have limitations. I hope to give enough information for YOU to decide if YOU would take aspirin if YOU were at high risk of a heart attack. I know I would!

STEVE was in his late 60s when he came to see me. He was slim, kept active and was generally well. This was his lipid profile:

	mg/dl	mmol/l	ideally
Total Cholesterol (TC)	**250**	5.6	< (less than) **200**/5.0
Triglycerides (TG)	**15**	0.4	<**80**/2.0
High Density Lipoprotein (HDL)	**95**	2.5	> (greater than) **40**/1.0
TC to HDL ratio		2.2	<4.0 ratio
Non HDL	**120**	3.1	<**155**/4.0
Low Density Lipoprotein (LDL)	**110**	2.9	<**95**/2.5

This looks fairly unremarkable. When I plugged his features into the Australian cardiovascular disease calculator, he had a risk of six percent of an event in five years. This is considered a low risk and was represented by a green bar.

He was concerned, however, because his brother, who was of similar build and without significant cardiac risk, had required by-pass grafting months earlier. Steve wanted to know if he were at risk. After we discussed

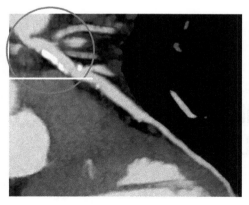

using cardiac CT imaging to obtain more information, Steve wished to proceed with the testing.

This image clearly demonstrates calcific (bright white) and non-calcific (dark) plaque. His calcium score was over 250 and, as can be seen from the image, there is significant plaque in the proximal part of the artery. My evaluation of the findings was that, left unattended, the plaque features suggested a greater than 20 percent risk of a cardiac event in 5 to 10 years, considerably higher than his risk calculator.

I spoke with Steve, reviewing his scan with him and explaining the

THE ULTIMATE MEMBERSHIP TO STAYING HEALTHY AND LIVING LONGER...

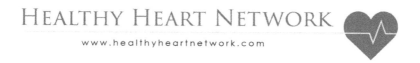

HEALTHY HEART NETWORK

www.healthyheartnetwork.com

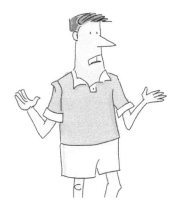

findings. My feeling was that the risk features were high enough to warrant consideration of statin therapy and aspirin, to modify risk.

He was happy to go on medication for prevention, together with his current healthy lifestyle. However, in Australia, his lipid profile didn't allow the prescription of a statin to be supported by the Pharmaceutical Benefits Scheme. This meant that he had to self-fund the medication which, with the information he then had, he was more than happy to do.

PENNY was 52 years old when she came to see me. She was generally well and on no medication. She was a non-smoker and didn't have elevated blood pressure. She was concerned, however, because she had a terrible family history of premature coronary disease. Her lipid profile was:

	mg/dl	mmol/l	ideally
Total Cholesterol (TC)	235	6.1	< (less than) **200**/ 5.0
Triglycerides (TG)	22	0.6	< **80**/ 2.0
High Density Lipoprotein (HDL)	80	2.1	> (greater than) **40**/ 1.0
TC to HDL ratio		2.1	<4.0 ratio
Non HDL	155	4.0	< **155**/ 4.0
Low Density Lipoprotein (LDL)	142	3.7	< **95**/ 2.5

If we put these results into the cardiovascular disease risk calculator, we see Penny's risk is estimated at one percent in five years and she gets a green indicator.

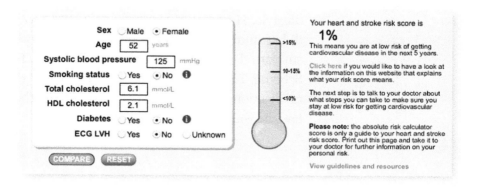

The important thing to remember here is that a risk calculator doesn't predict the risk for an **individual** patient. Rather, it provides the rate events occur in a **group** of 100 individuals with the same characteristics. This does not tell us who of the 100 will have the event.

Penny was well informed when she came to see me. She had already had a significant discussion with her general practitioner and had looked at my website to obtain information about scanning the heart. Her husband, who came with her, also decided to have his heart scanned. He was about the same age, with a similar lipid profile, had borderline blood pressure and had a bit of weight on his tummy. He was the one who looked as if he might have the unhealthy arteries.

This was Penny's calcium score image and results:

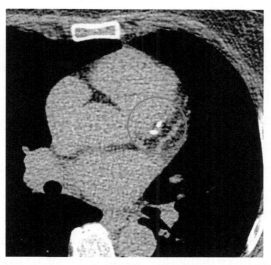

	Scoring Results : Agatston Score Protocol			
	LAD	LCX	RCA	Total Coronaries
Score	71.45	30.64	141.35	243.44
#ROI's	2	2	14	18
AreaSq (sq.mm.)	17.86	12.77	46.22	76.85

Her score of 243 is high for a young woman. For her age, the 90th percentile is 65! This result is three to four times higher, suggesting that Penny was probably the one out of 100, the one percent.

Although the results brought Penny to tears when she first heard this news, as the significance of having this knowledge sank in, she calmed down. There was no narrowing in the arteries and there had been no damage to the heart. And we had found what we had been looking for – to see if she had the same issues as others in her family. Although she did, **we had found the brake cylinder that was about to fail *before* the accident!**

We were able to institute therapy. For her, we were ahead of the game. There is little doubt that Penny found this process confronting but invaluable. And just to compete the story, her husband had a zero calcium score!

IMPORTANT POINTS

This series of patients includes examples of:

- high cholesterol and no evidence of problems in the arteries;
- high cholesterol and lots of plaque in the arteries;
- unremarkable lipid profile and high-risk features in the arteries, and
- family history with varying outcomes.

There is considerable complexity around these issues but I will discuss them in more detail throughout the book so that you will be equipped with the information you need to *Plan (not to have) Your Heart Attack.*

[1]   Cleland JG. Is aspirin useful in primary prevention? European heart journal 2013:eht287.

[2]   Nelson MR, Doust JA. Primary prevention of cardiovascular disease: new guidelines, technologies and therapies. Med J Aust 2013;198:606-10.

[3]   Berger JS, Brown DL, Becker RC. Low-dose aspirin in patients with stable cardiovascular disease: a meta-analysis. Am J Med 2008;121:43-9.

[4]   Collaborative meta-analysis of randomised trials of antiplatelet therapy for prevention of death, myocardial infarction, and stroke in high-risk patients. BMJ 2002;324:71-86.

The next chapter asks: "Is medical opportunity knocking on the door?" While there is no question that evidence-based medicine is the appropriate way to advance medical care, could rigid adherence to this approach hinder good medicine?

Chapter 4 -
The art of good medicine

> the discrepancy between evidence-based trials
and medical opportunity

Our discussion brings us to a point where there is an obvious medical opportunity to be ahead of the game in regard to an individual's coronary risk, by using a combination of the standard risk factor modelling and cardiac CT imaging. Why, then, is this not being done on a regular basis?

Cardiac CT imaging is not widely used in primary prevention because **no randomised double-blind control trials exist to demonstrate that it is beneficial in improving outcomes for the individuals who are scanned compared with a control group.** This is an absolutely critical point when it comes to understanding the slow uptake of a technology that would appear to be incredibly useful in the management of patients in a primary preventative role. The lack of clear-cut trial data means that there is a lack of an evidence base to support using cardiac CT imaging in primary prevention assessments.

Current medical practice, by and large, is founded on the concept of evidence-based medicine[1]. This means that patient management guidelines or recommendations which are put together by speciality groups or organisations are founded on a clear understanding that there has been appropriate research in an area and an unmistakable demonstration that the intervention being discussed has, without question, been shown to be beneficial.

There is absolutely **no question** that evidence-based medicine **is** the appropriate way to advance medical care. It is a solid foundation that demonstrates clearly that what we are doing has been proven to be safe and beneficial when applied to clinical practice[1]. All doctors need to be aware of the importance of evidence-based medicine in all undertakings in patient care. In no way should it be diminished.

Evidence-based limitations

While the importance of a body of evidence in any area of medicine helps to guide best practice and appropriate management for an individual, **sole reliance** on this approach presents potential limitations.

FIRSTLY, there is enormous complexity in medical/biological systems and sometimes multiple variables can be extremely difficult to assess in a large population over a long time.

For example, there is good evidence that aspirin is beneficial for patients who have had a myocardial infarction[2,3]. If, however, we were to ask, *Is it beneficial for patients who are left handed, wear spectacles and who are blond?* then, because those criteria were not necessarily tested during the trial, we would not have a definitive answer and, therefore, would not have a strong evidence base if we were dealing with a patient who was left handed, wore glasses and was blond. We would have to make an assumption and, as soon as we do that, by definition, we step away from evidence. This creates a rigidity to evidence-based medicine as it will never address all variables or questions in the evaluation of an individual with characteristics distinct from the average.

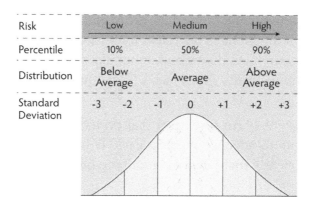

SECONDLY, the individual patient may be different to the evaluation of the averaged population from which the information has come. Populations will demonstrate a distribution curve which will have an average or mean but also have lower, as well as upper, extremes. The average results of the population may not be as applicable to the individuals at each end of the population spread. For example, we might undertake a study that gives us an average shoe size for adult males but is that applicable to our patient if he is a professional basketball player or a jockey?

THIRDLY, evidence-based medicine may have the limitation that the study has not been done and may never be done. This was highlighted in a paper published in the *British Medical Journal* in 2003 (Smith GC, Pell JP. *Parachute use to prevent death and major trauma related to gravitational challenge: systematic review of randomised controlled trials*[4]). It has affectionately become known as the "Parachute Paper".

In this paper the authors set out very clearly, within the appropriate and correct constructs of evidence-based medicine, that, **because of a clear lack of data** (specifically, randomised control trials surrounding the use of parachutes), **one can conclude that parachutes**

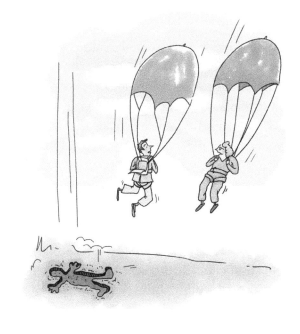

man: "Wow! What was that?"
woman: "Oh, that's Simon. First time jumper. Refused to use a parachute. Said there was no evidence that they worked!"

do not work. I believe the 'man on the street' quite happily accepts that parachutes do work. I think the 'man on the street' also accepts that it is not an absolute requirement for us to have a double-blind randomised control trial in which we would take a group of people with parachutes and push them out of a plane and then take, as the control group, another group of people without parachutes and push them out of a plane and compare the results!

This is a situation in which the randomised, double-blind controlled study has not been done. Common sense and, of course, an ethics committee, would never allow it to proceed. Clearly, it is a situation in which the observational data is reliable enough to draw a conclusion. However, it is an important reminder that **there will always be trials that have not been, and will not be, done and so there will be gaps in our evidence base within medicine.**

The first use of penicillin was so dramatic that its initial use was not randomised. The first 10 patients to receive an aortic valve (heart valve) replacement died before leaving hospital. This didn't stop the pursuit of a common sense solution to a clear problem. Further, there has never been a randomised controlled trial to assess the safety and efficacy of general anaesthesia. Think about it. Does general anaesthesia work? To find out, would you be prepared to be randomised in a study in which you could undergo surgery without anaesthesia? **The shortage of evidence-based studies did not stop these treatments from becoming commonly accepted.**

FOURTHLY, a study which has been undertaken to answer a question can, in retrospect, be seen to be **inadequately designed** and so does not fulfil all the requirements of its initial intention. This means that an evidence base can be constructed from research work which offers some, but not necessarily all, insight into a particular situation.

If I could illustrate this with an example. A study could be undertaken to look at the effect of reducing road accidents by reducing alcohol consumption. The study could be set up in controlled circumstances.

There may be one group who drinks alcohol and a control group who does not drink. This sounds like a very simple way to demonstrate that alcohol consumption would make a difference to the likelihood of a crash. The test could be undertaken on a regulated track and one would think that the data would clearly demonstrate that the individuals consuming alcohol would have a greater rate of accident.

Yet, if:

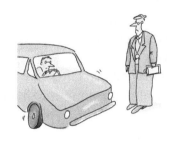

- all cars were limited to a top speed of 40km/hr because the investigators didn't want the risk of high speed accidents, and

- alcohol consumption were limited to one standard drink because the investigators were teetotallers and considered this a significant amount, then it is possible that the effect of alcohol on driving error may be significantly diminished by the slow speed and the low blood alcohol levels, such that the group who had consumed alcohol may not have a statistically significant increase of events compared with the control group.

If

- no speed limit were imposed;

- the participants were instructed to complete the track circuit as quickly as possible, and

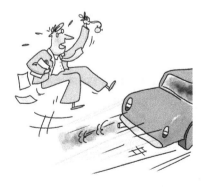

- they were instructed to drink to a blood alcohol level of greater than 0.05 percent (the legal limit in Australia), then there would be a clear difference due to the effect of alcohol.

In the above situation, the study design may actually lead to an outcome in which the full impact of an intervention (alcohol) is not appreciated statistically. The study may have been undertaken with meticulous attention to scientific rigour; it may have had unquestionable statistical analysis; it may tick all the required boxes to achieve merit for publication. This is very important because if this piece of information then forms part of the evidence base within that area of medicine, it brings with it the limitations of that trial design and results. In this situation, it would be possible to argue that under controlled conditions with good scientific rigour and extensive statistical analysis, alcohol was not shown to increase risk of accident. Only on looking deeper into the study would it become apparent that flaws with the study design (limiting speed and an inadequate alcohol consumption) might have lead to a misleading conclusion. Editorial comments during publication may flag these shortfalls but sometimes it is not until some time later that the limitation is recognised and the headline of the study remains to permeate more effectively than its detail.

This occurred with a major study designed specifically to demonstrate the value of cardiac CT imaging in risk assessment. The trial was called the St Francis Heart study[5]. The consequence of its failure has effectively applied a handbrake to the broader use of cardiac CT. I will discuss the study in more detail later *(refer to Chapter 16)*. Remember, also, that the best observational tool is the 'retro-spectroscope' and, in this situation, it is reasonable to expect that a study to explore a new area may not be designed as well as it could have been, because there was not enough knowledge at the time to guide the process.

FIFTHLY, time can erode 'evidence' in some situations as nothing stays the same. Think of the 'evidence' about mobile phones 20 years ago. Who would have said that most people would be carrying one now and more importantly, who would have imagined the functionality of smart phones today?

Time and changes in technology can move the goal posts in medicine, too. For example, when we advise patients that a new valve should last 15 years, what we are really saying is that valves that were made and implanted 20 plus years ago have been lasting around 15 years in the patients who received them. We can say that because it took a few years to become comfortable with the results, then time has been needed to track outcomes. What we don't really know is if the experience gained and the technology developed over the past 20 years mean that the valves currently being produced will last longer.

The same changing technology is impacting on CT imaging in regard to image quality. Radiation doses and even contrast doses are now out of date based on the leading-edge machines, which are improving with each tick of the clock and technological advance. This rapidly changing landscape of technology means it is very hard, almost impossible, to have robust 'current' data, as each time a study is started the new iteration of technology moves the goal posts again, and again, and again. This is good for the patient but not so good for having an evidence base that truly reflects an up-to-date situation.

PENULTIMATELY, studies can appear to provide conflicting information. Perhaps a recent trial proves the opposite results to a trial that we have relied on for some years. Which trial do we believe? Was the new one with better computing and technology more reliable or was the old trial more reliable?

This can be a difficult issue. In cardiology for example, niacin, or vitamin B3, has been used for many years to manage lipid levels in the blood. Some years ago, in a trial called the HATS[6] trial, niacin, together with a statin, showed significant outcome benefit. However, more recently, a trial called the AIM-HIGH[7] trial suggested niacin was not helpful and could be potentially harmful. The 'headline results' of the AIM-HIGH trial have thrown into question the role of niacin. I don't know the answer. The HATS trial was compelling in study design and outcome; the AIM-HIGH trial also had good design and interpretation. Where does that leave niacin?

LASTLY, there is the possibility that the results may not be reliable. There is a small chance that research, even from reputable institutions, may be under a cloud of suspicion. In 2010 it was discovered that an oncological researcher had manipulated the data in a number of his widely distributed papers to prove that a theory worked[8]. He was considered by many as being at the forefront of ovarian cancer research. He was based at the Duke University, considered an eminent medical institution[9]. This is one of the most significant cases in recent times[10]. However, there are more and no one knows how much impropriety is not detected. Where do vested interests intersect with funding proposals, publishing demands and a genuine and hopeful optimism to prove a truth, regardless of the results?

So, knowledge gaps, or evidence-free zones, have always and will always exist. It just is not possible to answer every question with every variable and then have the situation in which that can be applied to every individual, based on an averaged result that has been demonstrated in a population – assuming that is, that the right study was undertaken, with the right conduct.

Good medicine

In many ways, this represents the art of medicine and the reason why doctors will continue to exist, in spite of improving access to technology and information. **The role of an experienced medical practitioner is to evaluate the individual and that person's particular needs and then, knowing and being familiar with the evidence base and experience in other individuals, come to a conclusion which leads to an appropriate management plan**[1].

I try to explain this to my patients in a way that paints doctors a little like astronomers.

We look out into a universe that we do not fully understand, nor do we fully know its boundaries. Within that universe there are constellations, stars and moons. These are fixed points within that vast space that we have some certainty about. In medicine the fixed points are studies, trials that provide the 'evidence base'. When faced with an individual patient, it is our role to try to most appropriately fit our knowledge of that universe of information to the individual. It may be for a certain patient that we

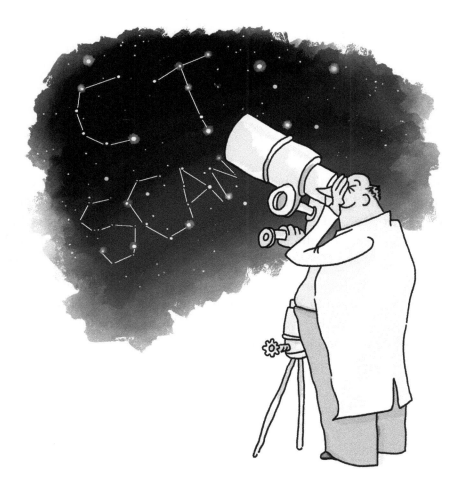

align those stars of knowledge into Orion. For another patient, we may rearrange those stars of knowledge to a different constellation, perhaps Capricorn or Aquarius, or the Big Dipper.

Being aware of where the evidence base lies is absolutely critical in appropriate care. It is also absolutely critical to be aware that the application of that evidence base has limitations and boundaries. It is our role to understand those boundaries as well as our patients and, through experience, try to find the best solution, the best answers and the best care for them.

Accepting their significance but, for the moment, putting aside the lack of evidence-based trials, what if we could identify patients who were going to have a heart attack soon and start primary prevention therapy before they have their coronary event?

This would require us to be far more precise in our evaluation of the **individual** and far less reliant on the risk of that individual within a **population.** What if in an intermediate-risk population, a group in which 15 people out of 100 will have an event in a 10 year period, we were able to find those 15 and start primary prevention therapy before their events?

While no formal, randomised study like this has been done (so it is an evidence-free zone) I put to you that, logically, it would seem that, if we can improve the way we find those high-risk people within the intermediate-risk population, then there is every chance we can make a meaningful difference.

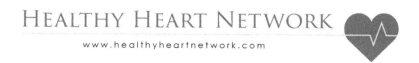

THE ULTIMATE MEMBERSHIP TO STAYING HEALTHY AND LIVING LONGER...

HEALTHY HEART NETWORK

www.healthyheartnetwork.com

IMPORTANT POINTS

- Current medical practice is founded on the concept of evidence-based medicine. This is the appropriate way to advance medical knowledge.

- However, sole reliance on this approach presents limitations, including:

  » the enormous complexities in medical/biological systems;

  » an individual patient may be different from the averaged population;

  » not all studies can be done, ethically and morally;

  » a study may be inadequately designed;

  » studies can appear to provide conflicting information, and

  » not all results are reliable.

- Medicine is like the universe: it is not fully understood nor are its boundaries accurately known. This leaves room for the 'art of medicine'.

[1] Sackett DL, Rosenberg WMC, Gray JAM, Haynes RB, Richardson WS. Evidence based medicine: what it is and what it isn't. BMJ 1996;312:71-72.

[2] Fang J, George MG, Gindi RM, et al. Use of low-dose aspirin as secondary prevention of atherosclerotic cardiovascular disease in US adults (from the National Health Interview Survey, 2012). The American Journal of Cardiology 2015;115:895-900.

[3] Collaborative meta-analysis of randomised trials of antiplatelet therapy for prevention of death, myocardial infarction, and stroke in high-risk patients. BMJ 2002;324:71-86.

[4] Smith GCS, Pell JP. Parachute use to prevent death and major trauma related to gravitational challenge: systematic review of randomised controlled trials. BMJ (Clinical research ed) 2003;327:1459-61.

[5]   Arad Y, Spadaro LA, Roth M, Newstein D, Guerci AD. Treatment of asymptomatic adults with elevated coronary calcium scores with atorvastatin, vitamin C, and vitamin E: the St. Francis Heart Study randomized clinical trial. J Am Coll Cardiol 2005;46:166-72.

[6]   Brown BG, Zhao XQ, Chait A, et al. Simvastatin and niacin, antioxidant vitamins, or the combination for the prevention of coronary disease. The New England journal of medicine 2001;345:1583-92.

[7]   Investigators A-H, Boden WE, Probstfield JL, et al. Niacin in patients with low HDL cholesterol levels receiving intensive statin therapy. The New England journal of medicine 2011;365:2255-67.

[8]   Rothschild D, Biggest Offender of Medical Research Misconduct in History? 2012. Feb 16, 2012 4:11:00 PM
(Accessed at http://www.ithenticate.com/plagiarism-detection-blog/bid/78874 Biggest-Offender-of-Medical-Research-Misconduct-in-History#.Vo5a9_l95hF.)

[9]   Pelley S, Deception at Duke. CBS News, 2012. February 12th, 2012 (Accessed at http://www.cbsnews.com/8301-18560_162-57376073/deception-at-duke/.)

[10]   Oransky I, The Anil Potti retraction record so far. Retraction Watch, 2012. February 14th, 2012
(Accessed at http://retractionwatch.wordpress.com/2012/02/14the-anil-potti-retraction-record-so-far/.)

In the next chapter we consider new possibilities for preventative cardiology.

A personal approach to managing the individual rather than the population in an attempt to stop a heart attack before it occurs

The remainder of the book reflects my approach to primary prevention of coronary artery disease or stopping a heart attack before it occurs. I offer it to you in an effort to bring as much information as possible to the appropriate management of an individual, understanding the lack of a clear-cut evidence base but drawing from observational data, common sense and the 'art of medicine'.

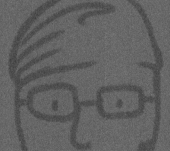

Dr Warrick Bishop is an experienced cardiologist with extensive training and expertise in the area of CT coronary angiography. His very proactive approach to cardiac health has been an integral part of his methodology throughout his career. Having known Warrick for 25 years, I can assure you it is not a recent fashionable trend. His practice has always been and remains very focussed on 'best care' for individual cardiac patients as he takes a holistic approach to patient management.

Alistair Begg, cardiologist, Adelaide

Chapter 5 -
Image is everything

> medical and technological advances that
make possible new opportunities for primary
preventative cardiology

A key element to any new approach to primary prevention and risk assessment is the availability of, and accessibility to, imaging the coronary arteries using CT scanning. This is a non-invasive, safe way to evaluate the build-up of cholesterol, or atheroma, to give an indication of the health of the coronary arteries in an asymptomatic person. Central to this, we must understand that a build-up of cholesterol within the arteries generally leads to **associated deposits of calcium** in the artery, so that calcium can be used as an indicator of plaque build-up.

Calcium

For more than 80 years, observations have been made, primarily by radiologists in the earlier years, that calcium could build up in the arteries, although there were differing opinions about its significance.

As far back as 1930 observations were made by German physician R. Lenk[1] in an article, "Rontgendiagnose der koronarsklerose in vivo", that calcium could be detected in the coronary arteries of "living subjects". This was reported again in 1959 in the United States by D. H. Blankenhorn and D. Stearne[2] who, using x-rays on cadavers, demonstrated the presence of calcification within the coronary arteries. About the same time, in the United Kingdom, M. F. Oliver and his colleagues[3] used fluoroscopy (or rapid acquisition x-ray to allow assessment during movement) to assess coronary artery disease using calcium as an indicator of potential problems in living subjects.

A study by McGuire in 1968[4] looked at calcification within the coronary arteries in patients who had had symptoms of angina or who had had a heart attack compared with a control group who had had no known problems. This simple study, which evaluated several hundred people, suggested that the development of calcification within the coronary arteries may be a useful guide or indicator of risk in an individual. The summary from that study is:

Five hundred and forty-four unselected patients were examined by a radiologist to determine the presence or absence of coronary artery calcification. The overall incidence of coronary calcification was 20 percent and there was a definite increase in the frequency of the finding with increasing age. A comparison of 94 patients with coronary calcification with a matched control group, without calcification, indicated that the prevalence of symptomatic ischaemic heart disease in the group with calcification was approximately twice that of the control group. The correlation was even more significant when the degree of calcification was moderate or severe. (Ischaemic heart disease is reduced blood supply to the heart.)

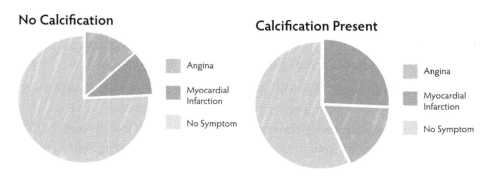

The McGuire study shows that the more green, the better. It is easy to see that the presence of calcification is associated with less green.

Although this observational study was undertaken almost 50 years ago, it is engaging in terms of suggesting the possibility that imaging of the coronary arteries could be a valuable indicator of the risk an individual patient carries. Although this early work was interesting and potentially tantalising in the opportunities it offered, it was not really picked up. This is probably because the process used high amounts of x-ray radiation, was limited by the availability of fluoroscopy and offered limited quantification of the findings, which were described as "not present", "mild", "moderate" or "severe".

It was not until the 1980s when a technology called **electron beam computed tomography** (EBCT) became available that interest was again ignited in trying to evaluate the health of an individual's coronary arteries. EBCT simply means that, using enormous magnets, x-rays are deflected at very high speed to acquire images which are then reconstructed, giving rise to the term **computed tomography** (CT). In the 1980s EBCT scanners were large and extremely expensive and only a few machines existed worldwide.

It is important to understand that imaging the heart has always been difficult because the heart moves and so any method of imaging needs to be extremely fast.

An American cardiologist, Arthur Agatston, realised a potential value in imaging or scanning the heart arteries to make an assessment of the amount of calcium within them, to potentially aid in risk assessment. Agatston published his work in 1990 and the **Agatston Score** has become a standardised method of evaluating the coronary arteries for the presence of calcification[5]. The score uses three millimetre slices (defined by the EBCT specifications) through the heart and then a combination of volume and density of the calcium detected to generate a number or 'score'.

In 1996, a pathologist, J. A. Rumberger, established the clear relationship between calcium and cholesterol within the structure of atheromatous plaque. Rumberger showed that **calcium moved into**

the wall of the artery following the deposition of cholesterol and then scavenger cells, with subsequent formation of scar tissue within a plaque[6].

This is an important point that I make to my patients. Calcium acts as a *marker* of the process with which we are concerned, that is, the presence of atherosclerotic plaque within the arteries.

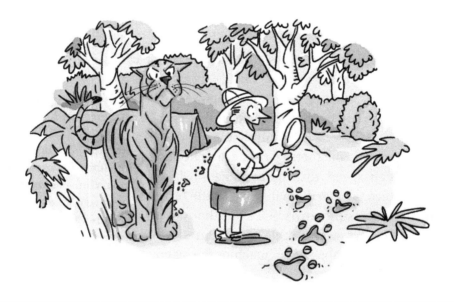

Calcium is the tiger's footprint and atheroma is the tiger.

Often patients will ask, "What can we do to get rid of the calcium?" but calcium is not the issue. **Calcium is simply the surrogate marker we use to give an indication of the process we are concerned about, the build-up of plaque within the coronary arteries.** I use the example that if, on pitching a tent in the jungle, we saw lots of tiger foot prints, it would mean that tigers are around and it might not be a great place to pitch the tent. Not seeing tiger foot prints doesn't mean there are not tigers in the area but it certainly makes it a better place to pitch a tent.

The calcium is a bystander, not the problem. Calcium itself is fairly inert in arteries, so it can stay there. We are wanting to deal with the process that put it there.

....

Supplements

Patients often are already taking a calcium supplement and/or vitamin D, and are concerned about whether or not they should continue. The jury is still out on this[7].

There is inconclusive data in relation to supplementation and coronary calcification. My general recommendation, however, is that if there are significant issues with the bones (osteoporosis or 'thin bones') such that supplementation is indicated, then supplementation should be considered.

If there are no clear issues with the bones I suggest that vitamin D is probably best taken by sun exposure to the skin. There is no naturally occurring oral form of vitamin D (and remember, some oral dosages can lead to levels far higher than seen physiologically). Similarly, I suggest dietary calcium (cheese, dairy, meat, yoghurt) is also the most natural way. By virtue of the amount of calcium contained in them, taking tablets will lead to levels of calcium in the bloodstream that are far greater than would be seen in nature. This is best avoided, I suggest, until we know more about it.

....

CT technology evolution

CT technology has moved on a long way since the 1980s and 90s. Since about 2006, a new generation of CT machines has become available. These machines are smaller, faster, cheaper and use the same or less radiation than the original EBCT scanners.

Today's CT scanners image the heart using a gantry system (a large ring) that spins x-ray heads and detectors around the patient at high speed. Each rotation of image acquisition can obtain from four centimetres to the full vertical distance of the heart. The speed of rotation is very fast, and continues to increase with improvements in technology. Because the heart is constantly moving, the faster the image can be acquired, the less blur and the better quality of the image. This is similar to using fast shutter speeds on regular cameras to take action photographs. These new machines, with more detectors and faster rotation times, are being used with advanced technologies that reduce the radiation doses to below ordinary yearly background radiation.

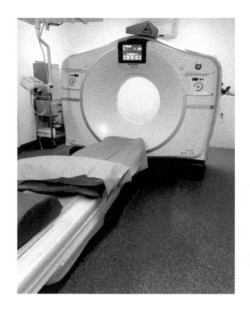

This means that our current technology is able to **accurately, reliably** and **reproducibly** acquire images of the arteries of the heart for evaluation of calcification. The current generation of machines is validated to apply the score generated by Agatston et al[8].

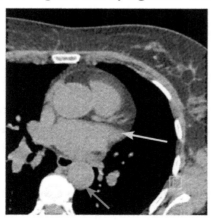

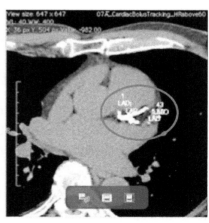

This is an image of zero calcium score. The yellow arrow points to the heart; the red arrow to the aorta.

This is an image showing extensive calcification of the left anterior descending artery and circumflex artery.

Along with increased speed, improved image acquisition and the reduction of the radiation dose, there has been increasing interest in injecting contrast into the vein in a patient's arm and then tracking that contrast through the body, into the arteries of the heart, to then outline the arteries. This is called a **coronary computed tomography angiogram** or a CCTA, often referred to as a CT coronary angiogram.

Further to showing the presence of calcium, **CT coronary angiography outlines the coronary artery in exquisite detail**, giving information about the location of plaque, the quality and nature of the plaque, degree of stenosis and size of vessel affected. **This information had previously not been obtainable, non-invasively, in a living patient.**

The development of this technology, together with the development of protocols for imaging, both of calcium within the arteries and tracing contrast through the arteries to outline specific detail, are major changes in what is available when assessing the coronary arteries and a patient's risk potential. This combined imaging of coronary calcium scoring and CT coronary angiography provides an opportunity to make an evaluation of an individual patient's arteries and the patient's individual risk, as opposed to what the risk may be in a population of patients with similar risk factors.

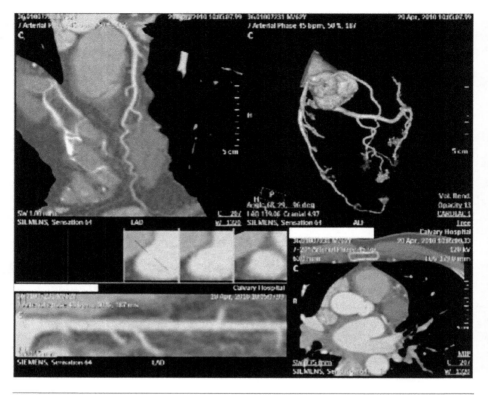

This image shows the amazing detail of a CT coronary angiogram. This is the information available to the doctor reviewing or reporting a CCTA on a specially dedicated workstation.

The top left is the artery isolated within the other chest structures.
The top right is the 3D reconstruction of the patient's coronary tree.
The bottom right is the horizontal slices through the chest, also called axials.
The bottom left is called a spindle view and is the artery stretched out straight
and can be spun on its axis.
These images are too complex to cover in this discussion but
you can appreciate the fantastic pictures we can see.

IMPORTANT POINTS

- Calcium has been observed in the arteries of living subjects for more than 80 years. Over time this has become standardised with the use of the Agatston Score during non-contrast CT imaging.

- More recently, technology has improved and now dye/contrast can be injected during a CT scan to outline the coronary arteries in exquisite detail.

- Combining non-contrast and contrast CT imaging of the heart gives previously unobtainable information about the coronary arteries that can add to the risk assessment of an individual.

[1] Lenk R. Rontgendiagnose der Koronarsklerose in vivo. Fortschr ad Geb d 1927.

[2] Blankenhorn DH, Stern D. Calcification of the coronary arteries. Am J Roentgenol Radium Ther Nucl Med 1959;81:772-7.

[3] Oliver MF, Samuel E, Morley P, Young GB, Kapur PL. Detection of Coronary-Artery Calcification during Life. Lancet 1964;1:891-5.

[4] McGuire J, Chou TC, Schneider HJ. Visualization of calcification of the coronary arteries by the image intensifier. Transactions of the American Clinical and Climatological Association 1968;79:61-66.

[5] Agatston AS, Janowitz WR, Hildner FJ, Zusmer NR, Viamonte M, Jr., Detrano R. Quantification of coronary artery calcium using ultrafast computed tomography. J Am Coll Cardiol 1990;15:827-32.

[6] Wexler L, Brundage B, Crouse J, et al. Coronary Artery Calcification: Pathophysiology, Epidemiology, Imaging Methods, and Clinical Implications: A Statement for Health Professionals From the American Heart Association. Circulation 1996;94:1175-92.

[7] Manson JE, Allison MA, Carr JJ, et al. Calcium/vitamin D supplementation and coronary artery calcification. Menopause (New York, NY) 2010;17:683.

[8] Schmermund A, Erbel R, Silber S. Age and gender distribution of coronary artery calcium measured by four-slice computed tomography in 2,030 persons with no symptoms of coronary artery disease. American Journal of Cardiology;90:168-73.

Cardiac CT imaging's ability to evaluate the extent of cholesterol build-up before the onset of a problem is discussed more fully in the next chapter.

Chapter 6 -
Changing times, changing terminology

> what is a disease before it is a disease?
coronary atheroma burden

> risk factors vs localised findings

The ability for cardiac CT imaging to demonstrate the presence of atheroma or plaque within the arteries is a paradigm shift in the conventional management of coronary artery disease.

As discussed earlier, historically, coronary artery disease has been diagnosed at the time of the event, the time a patient has had chest pain, shortness of breath or a major adverse coronary event. By that time, the patient has developed a 'disease' which simply means a symptom or loss of normal function.

Changing terminology

I have patients who undergo cardiac CT imaging for risk evaluation and in whom we demonstrate the presence of plaque build-up. These are otherwise healthy patients looking to maximise their primary prevention strategies. **This is the exciting opportunity that cardiac CT imaging offers; it gives us an ability to evaluate the extent of plaque build-up *before* the onset of a problem.** Intuitively, one might think this is extremely valuable in the process of attempting to evaluate the potential risk that an individual may carry in regard to the development of coronary artery disease. Yet, although cardiac CT imaging has been readily available for the past 5 to 10 years, there has been no clear consensus for the description of plaque formation prior to the occurrence of symptoms or loss of function, to describe the 'pre-disease state'.

In these cases, I do not feel comfortable calling formation of plaque in the arteries 'coronary artery disease' before an event or problem, and in a patient without any symptoms. There are four reasons why I specifically avoid the term 'disease' in describing plaque formation found on scanning **before** a patient has had any problems.

1. *It is not yet a disease.* As the patient has not experienced any event or symptom, the term 'disease' is not well received by the patient. It is much easier to have the conversation around a "build-up of cholesterol in the arteries that needs management", than label the patient as having a 'disease'. There is significant psychological cost in diagnosing a 'disease' particularly in a patient who has presented in a primary preventive capacity, and is otherwise feeling well. My objective, as a preventative cardiologist, is to keep that patient healthy and well, with the goal being to avoid the development of 'disease'.

2. *Coronary artery disease, as a term, has no variation or scope of degree that can be applied to it.* It is binary; it is either present or not. If we are looking at someone who has a build-up of plaque in the arteries, it could be severe, minimal or somewhere in between. This subtlety or gradation of severity is not conveyed in the term 'coronary artery disease'.

3. *Cholesterol deposition within the arteries appears to be part of the ageing process.* If any of us were to live long enough we would all have evidence of wear and tear within our coronary arteries. The final common result of this would be the development of atheromatous plaque. That this occurs more rapidly in some people simply reflects individual predisposition and does not necessarily reflect the early stages of a 'disease state'. If we accept ageing as a natural process and we accept wear and tear as a natural process, then the development of cholesterol deposition and plaque formation within the arteries is on that spectrum. Early in the process, it is simply a predisposition and does not warrant the label 'disease'. A parallel example might be someone who has a 'clicky' hip or a 'clicky' knee which, in many

years to come, *may* lead to arthritic change and eventually require the replacement of an arthritic joint. However, in the early stages, it is simply showing signs of wear and tear, or features consistent with ageing.

4. *The label of coronary artery disease has immediate and rigid implications in situations such as insurance or licensing,* situations that may lead to a knee jerk response or reaction without attention to gradation or severity, resulting in a misdirected or disproportionate response.

The term I use with patients and in correspondence in a primary preventative setting, to describe finding plaque within the arteries in a patient who is otherwise well, is **coronary atheroma burden.** This is a description for the **extent of plaque formation within the coronary arteries as demonstrated on imaging before the development of disease.** The use of this terminology then allows more precision around the description of the cardiac CT findings, such that a patient may demonstrate low-risk atheroma burden, high-risk atheroma burden or something in between. *(I explore this concept in more detail in my book "Have You Planned Your Heart Attack?")*

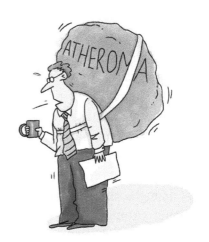

Changing our understanding

The other significant observation is that as we image coronary arteries in a primary prevention role, we are discovering that **the plaque formation can be very localised.** The interesting thing about this is that our risk factor model for the evaluation of the likely development of a problem with coronary artery disease focusses on factors which affect the whole body: age, cholesterol, blood pressure, diabetes, smoking, diet and exercise. One could think these factors would also affect a coronary artery equally – but they do not!

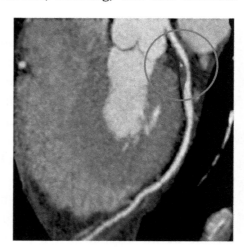

Imaging clearly demonstrates that plaque formation may occur in only one or two locations within the coronary artery tree. This means that an individual's future may be defined by a single plaque that is little more than a centimetre in length. Remembering that the main branches of the coronary arteries are 35-40cm in combined total length, this is a small fraction of the coronary tree, yet it may determine a life or death outcome for the patient.

This scan shows one large life-threatening proximal plaque in the left anterior descending artery. The remainder of the LAD and the other vessels in this patient were clear of plaque.

This means that there is an interplay between local factors within the artery and the risk factors which the individual may have:

- traditional risk factors, based on observational studies over many years, clearly indicate that certain cardiovascular risk factors are important associations in the development of coronary artery disease in an individual, and

- there is no question that there are local features within an individual's arteries that may potentially be regulated by these more general risk factors.

The complexity of this is that there are people who have what would be considered high-level cardiovascular risk factors and yet there are no local features within their arteries and no development of plaque.

Conversely, there may be patients who have low or intermediate cardiovascular risk factors but significant local predisposition in their arteries, showing substantial or high risk atheroma burden.

The only way we can sensibly deal with this situation, in my opinion, is to understand that **our prediction based on risk factors alone is only part of the puzzle.** This may be accurate for dealing with large populations but falls short for the individual when we have no mechanism for assessing local factors within the artery.

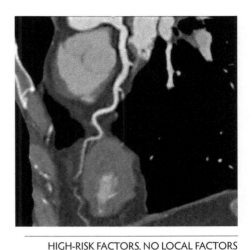

HIGH-RISK FACTORS, NO LOCAL FACTORS
This patient was a 62-year-old male with the following lipid profile:
TC 9.1, TG 3.3, HDL 1.5, Ratio 6.6, LDL 6.6.
He had also been non-insulin dependant diabetic for five years. Surprisingly, there is no evidence of atheroma burden.

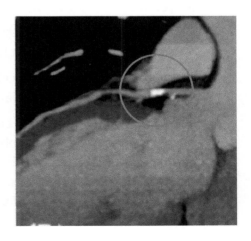

It is with this background that the role of imaging the arteries in an individual begins to make more sense.

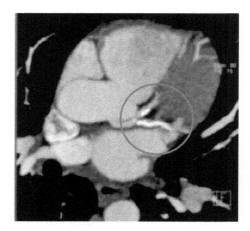

AVERAGE RISK FACTORS, SIGNIFICANT LOCAL FACTORS

This well 48-year-old male had no diabetes and a lipid profile of TC 5.8, HDL 1.1, TG 1.3 (unremarkable). He undertook very regular exercise, was not over-weight, had no family history, no hypertension and did not smoke. The scan shows surprisingly extensive atheroma burden.

IMPORTANT POINTS

- Cardiac CT reveals the extent and distribution of plaque in the arteries.

- 'Disease' is defined by symptoms or loss of function.

- 'Coronary artery disease' refers to the complications (symptoms or loss of function) from build-up of cholesterol in the arteries.

- Cholesterol build-up **before** a problem occurs is perhaps best referred to as **atheroma burden** as it has not yet become a 'disease'.

- Plaque burden can be very localised, suggesting that local factors within the artery must also play a role in plaque development.

- Combining non-contrast and contrast cardiac CT imaging of the heart gives previously unobtainable information about the coronary arteries. Atheroma burden can be assessed in relation to its location and before complications arise. This can aid risk assessment and management for the individual.

Common scenarios that present for cardiovascular risk management are highlighted in the next chapter.

Chapter 7 -
What about my arteries?

> common investigative scenarios

General practitioners (GPs) refer to me to assist in particular situations of cardiovascular risk management for their patients. Due to my belief in the investigative value of the technology and the process, and having been involved in the establishment of a cardiac CT service for the local region, I have developed a particular interest in cardiac CT imaging and related information that help in decisions around future risk and patient management. I have been involved in the assessment, preparation, reading of the study and interpretation of the findings, and then the application of that information to individual patients in close to 3000 cases. The most common scenarios I deal with are patients who don't want to take statins or they are intolerant of them, there is a family history of heart problems or they want reassurance.

"I don't want to take statins"

I often see patients with high risk factors who do not want to take statins, drugs that can lower cholesterol in the blood. In recent years there has been significant media interest and comment surrounding the role of statins, causing confusion and

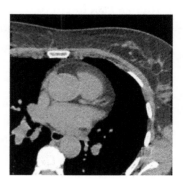

This is a zero calcium score in a 66-year-old active female who had worked hard on lifestyle modification for three years as she wanted to avoid statin therapy. She had a total cholesterol of 8.8, triglyceride of 1.3, a high density lipoprotein of 2.0 and a low density lipoprotein of 6.6 with a ratio of 4.4. Fasting glucose was 5.1 and she had been started on 20mg of rosuvastatin (a statin) by her GP. With a zero score, the literature suggests that her risk of a MACE in the next 10 years is less than one percent. This is the case, even with her high cholesterol levels.

uncertainty concerning their benefits, as well as raising questions about possible side-effects. There are many patients who have been started on cholesterol-lowering agents by their GP, in the context of cardiovascular risk, but who would rather not be on a medication, unless that medication were absolutely necessary.

Intolerant of statins

I also see patients with high cholesterol levels and high-risk features but who are intolerant of statins. Both patients and GPs manifest a sense of frustration as there is difficulty in achieving appropriate cholesterol targets in an individual who, with elevated cholesterol and a perceived high risk, is intolerant of the agent. The reason for the referral to me is for an evaluation to produce extra information that could provide more guidance in terms of the individual's needs.

The questions being asked are: *What is going on in the arteries? Is this patient's risk really as high as imagined? Is there evidence of significant plaque build-up in the arteries? Does this patient need to persist with the statins and be more accepting of (mild to moderate) side-effects? Could this patient be managed on a lower dose of statin? Is this patient's risk likely to be low, given there is minimal or no clear evidence of coronary cholesterol build-up? Perhaps the perceived risk, which is a population-based risk, is not accurate for this individual?*

....

I discuss the balance between traditional risk factor prediction and the cardiac CT risk in a user guide for doctors in appendix 3 of my book "Have You Planned Your Heart Attack?"

....

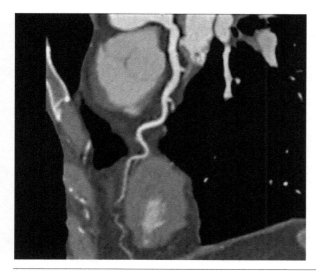

This is a cardiac CT image of a 62-year-old male who is statin intolerant. His total cholesterol was 9.1, his triglyceride was 3.3, his high density lipoprotein was 1.5, his low density lipoprotein was 6.6 and his total cholesterol to HDL ratio was 6.6. He had been a non-insulin dependent diabetic for five years. He had tried every statin given at high doses because of his cholesterol level and each had given him liver abnormality. He was a non-smoker, with normal blood pressure and no family history of premature coronary artery disease. He had no symptoms. The cardiac CT showed negligible or very low-risk atheroma build-up.

This patient's risk factors cannot be ignored. However, the finding of low-risk features (almost nothing!) in his arteries means that, at least in the short to intermediate term, his risks are much lower than predicted from risk calculation. This may then allow the introduction of a statin at lower doses, in an effort to avoid the liver side-effects, and an acceptance that treating to strict targets may not be immediately critical.

Family history of heart problems

I see numerous patients who have a significant family history of premature coronary artery disease (male younger than 55 years old or female younger than 60 years old who has had a MACE) but who seem to have relatively low- or intermediate-risk features, based on standard cardiovascular risk calculation. These patients come, knowing that there has been the loss of family members at a young age, unexpectedly and, understandably, very traumatically. These patients, quite reasonably, want to know if they are at the same risk. It is often the case that standard cardiovascular risk calculators do not include family history as one of the variables and so, young patients, particularly with concerning family histories, are often poorly risk-categorised by standard risk calculators.

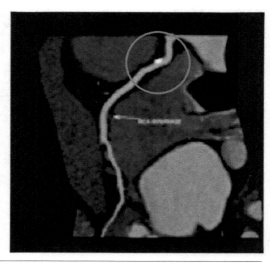

This is the cardiac CT of a 42-year-old male whose father died aged 51 and whose grandfather died at 53. The man's lipid profile was completely unremarkable, with a total cholesterol to high density lipoprotein ratio of 4 and normal triglycerides. He played competitive sport and was a smoker. The cardiac CT clearly shows early plaque formation at the beginning of the right coronary artery. After the scan, the patient started appropriate risk management therapy and quit smoking.

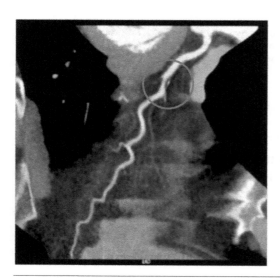

This is the CT angiogram of a 65-year-old exploration geologist with an untidy lipid profile and a lifestyle not conducive to good healthy habits. Travelling to places like the Congo, Peru and outback Australia, he wanted to know if he was going to have a heart attack in some remote far-flung region of the world. With these findings of high-risk plaque in the LAD, we were able to implement therapy to reduce his risk of event and increase the chance of his returning home safely after his trips away.

"I just want to know"

The final group consists of those in the low- to intermediate-risk group who simply want some clarity for themselves around risk. They may have borderline blood pressure, carry a little extra weight, exhibit borderline cholesterol levels, don't exercise as much as they think they should. However, they have seen friends, colleagues or loved ones who were seemingly well and not obviously at increased risk, have coronary events or die. These people are seeking some clarity and certainty around their personal risk, rather than the risk that may be attributable to a population with similar characteristics.

IMPORTANT POINTS

- Common scenarios point to the complexities and variations that build further support for the premise that knowing the individual's **actual** situation is greatly preferable for treatment, management and reassurance than relying on population-based averages.

Let's have a detailed look at the role of calcium as an indicator of potential risk.

Chapter 8 -
Evaluating and reporting risk

Today's approach to risk evaluation is, in general terms, related to evaluating factors that have been shown to be associated with increased risk in population studies and then applied to the individual: factors such as age, smoking, presence or absence of diabetes, cholesterol levels. These are the risk factor associations that give rise to **possible** development of a problem based on the observations associated with major adverse coronary events in large population studies.

For the sake of this discussion, I will refer to these risk factors as **'traditional'** risk factors and I will introduce a separate concept, **'plaque-**specific' risk. By this, I mean that there are features which are demonstrated on cardiac CT imaging, particularly relating to the plaque in question. The individual plaque (or plaques) may have a clear and specific impact on the risk of the potential development of a major adverse coronary event but, importantly, the risk is plaque-specific and may not necessarily match up with the risk suggested by the traditional risk factors.

It is important to understand that **both are significant and should be used in combination** in the decision-making related to the best ongoing care and risk modification of an individual patient.

Currently, **there is no standardised, structured approach to the description of risk within cardiac CT imaging.** For previously discussed historical reasons, the emphasis of risk association and imaging of the heart have been principally the domain of calcium scoring, which provides an indicator of the propensity of an individual patient to develop coronary atheroma within the arteries. In this regard, coronary calcification could be considered as a **traditional** risk indicator. This is particularly so with higher range calcium scores. Progressing to CT coronary angiography (the injection of contrast to outline the lumen of the artery, thus providing detail about the structure of individual plaques) gives an opportunity to make an assessment that relates to **plaque**-specific risk.

Regardless of a patient's cholesterol levels, the amount of exercise he or she undertakes (or not), how healthy the person claims his or her diet is, I want to know the health of **that** individual's arteries, not the risk that a population of people with the same characteristics may have. To do this, I believe, we get the most information by using CT to look directly at the arteries.

Coronary calcium score and risk

My practice is to obtain a coronary calcium score. Calcium scoring provides a sensitive indicator to the presence of atheroma. It is an absolute number and there is a significant body of research which supports the premise that the greater the absolute coronary calcium score, then the greater the risk of an event that an individual carries.

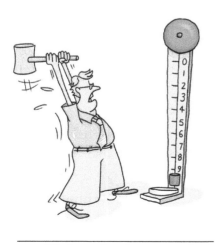

Who knows what calcium score you'll get?

As we have already discussed, **calcium is not the problem** but is an indicator of a potential risk. **The problem is the plaque build-up.** Scavenger cells, the macrophages, try to clean up the cholesterol and, in so doing so, can become so 'full' that they burst and spill their contents which include digestive enzymes. The enzymes cause scarring in the artery wall. The build-up of cholesterol, scavenger cells, scar tissue and calcium in the wall of the artery is the plaque. Agatston's early work in demonstrating an association between the amount of calcium present in an individual's arteries and the risk of progressing to a major adverse coronary event means that calcium scoring has become a prominent and sensible marker in risk assessment.

Observational data in relation to people with a zero calcium score is robust. It covers more than 30,000 patients and indicates that a zero calcium score carries a less than one percent chance of a coronary event in a 10 year period[1-3]. This makes **coronary calcium scoring a very powerful negative predictive test** (meaning the condition is not present) in cardiology. Neither a normal stress test (running on a treadmill), nor a normal invasive coronary angiogram (when contrast or dye is injected directly down the arteries) can provide the same assurance, while 'low cholesterol', 'regular exercise', 'good diet', 'watching my weight' and a 'healthy lifestyle' cannot come anywhere near to being as useful in predicting a low risk of an event as does a zero coronary calcium score.

....

This next section is controversial and may cause a negative response from my colleagues who are ardent practitioners of evidence-based medicine and advocates of guidelines. Some of my colleagues, however, will see a line of logic that stitches together patches of evidence where gaps exist.

For patients, I hope it provides information that can form the basis of a sensible discussion with their medical practitioners, in order to meet their own particular needs.

....

Calcium as a gatekeeper

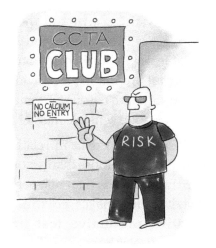

Due to this robust body of data, my own practice is to use the coronary calcium score (CCS) in its own right or as a gatekeeper to CT coronary angiography. My feeling is that not everyone needs both a calcium score and a CT coronary angiogram for risk stratification.

If, however, an abnormality is detected, then it **is** my general recommendation that we progress to CT coronary angiography, to obtain as much information as possible about the health of that patient's coronary arteries.

Current literature and guidelines support the use of CCS alone for risk stratification, particularly for intermediate-risk patients[4].

My own experience, however, is that in certain patients the amount of calcium underestimates the actual plaque burden present. This tends to be the case in younger patients who may have a family history of premature coronary disease, perhaps with elevated triglycerides and non-HDL cholesterol, features of insulin resistance (increased waist to hip ratio) or even a family history of type 2 diabetes. In these cases, the CCS may be low but this may be in the setting of a large non-calcific (cholesterol dominant) plaque burden, such that the patient is likely to carry a much higher risk of a MACE than suggested by the CCS alone.

Until we have clear information from the literature that tells us reliably how to identify those patients, their risk is significantly underestimated by the CCS alone. I'm comfortable with explaining this situation to the patient and allowing the patient to be involved in calcium scoring alone, or calcium scoring followed by CCTA if calcium is present.

Why not CCTA for everyone?

To use a coronary calcium score only has several benefits.

FIRSTLY, in the asymptomatic patient, the literature supports that a zero score is a very reassuring test.

SECONDLY, it provides a lower radiation dose than a cardiac CT (CCS + CCTA) study. At every stage in medicine we need to be asking the question: Is the risk of a particular test outweighed by its benefit? With a low radiation dose from calcium scoring resulting in a zero calcium score, there seems to be little point in subjecting the patient to further radiation when the negative predictive value of a zero calcium score is so low.

THIRDLY, it is a relatively cheap test. Why progress to a more expensive test when the first has already demonstrated a very low risk over the next 10 years?

FOURTHLY, the coronary calcium score requires no contrast, is extremely safe and avoids any potential risk or complication associated with the injection of contrast media or dye.

Importantly, in this setting of asymptomatic patient evaluation, there is no data to suggest that CCTA adds incremental information in risk stratification over and above the CCS. In fact, there is published literature that suggests adding CCTA to CCS adds no benefit[5]. The limitation of that data, however, is that it is observational data from a registry that was not a dedicated study to explore the possible additional benefit of adding CCTA information to CCS information in management and then outcome. Only the degree of stenosis was used rather than including other features of plaque *(discussed later)* that may have added to more precision and a different outcome. Also, there is some data from the same group suggesting that *there is incremental outcome prediction benefit* in adding CCTA to CCS in patients with symptoms[6].

My experience is that if we find calcium on the CCS then, unless we follow up with the CCTA, it is not possible to be clear as to the health of that individual's arteries. *(I discuss this approach in more detail for medical practitioners in Appendix 3)*

There is one other specific practice I have surrounding coronary calcium scoring and that is using fine cut (0.6mm) sections in men who are under 50 years of age and women under 60. Remember, the standard Agatston Score uses three millimetre slices (set by the specifications of the scanner)[7]. So, I'm talking about using thinner slices (available on the modern machines, which were not available to Agatston for his original work) to look at the heart to be more precise in the detection of calcifications.

Coronary calcuim score and coronary event risk (CER)

	10 YEAR CER		
Baseline coronary calcium score	With diabetes	With metabolic syndrome	With neither diabetes nor metabolic syndrome
0	2.0%	0.8%	0.6%
1-99	8.8%	5.5%	3.5%
100-399	14.5%	12.5%	6.3%
400 or more	16.9%	15.8%	11.3%

Data from average 4-6 year follow-up of patients in the Multi-Ethnic Study of Atherosclerosis (MESA). Dr Malik. Jan 2010.

I use the fine cut because small amounts of calcium may be present that could relate to a build-up of plaque, yet might not be picked up on standard Agatston scoring in which the speck of calcium may not be big enough to register. A zero score in this situation could be erroneous[8]. The likelihood of this misleading zero score becomes less as the patient gets older[9].

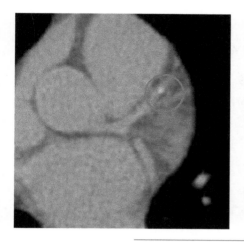 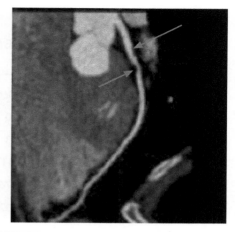

This scan shows a fleck of calcium on the left (a zero score) and the significant cholesterol build-up that was associated with it in a male under 50 years of age.

Sex and age

As a person ages, that person is more likely to have some evidence of calcium within the arteries. This brings us to the concept of an expected CCS score range for age and sex, or a percentile score for age and sex. It poses the question: *What's an average calcium score for my age and sex?*

Within each age and sex population, there is a distribution. For example, in a group of one hundred 50-year-old-men, the lowest risk 25 men will have a zero calcium score (this is the lowest quarter of scores and called "first quartile"), while the highest risk 25 men will have scores of over 100 (this is called the "fourth quartile"). *(Please refer to the coronary calcium score percentile chart on right[10].)*

By using men at 50 and women at 60 as the cut-off for zero Agatston scores, I am ensuring that a zero calcium score represents the best quartile for that age/sex group and so may not be inadvertently representing a higher risk *(see circles on chart).*

Coronary calcuim score percentile chart

	AGE (Years)						
	35–39	40–44	45–49	50–54	55–59	60–64	65–70
Men	(479)	(859)	(1066)	(1085)	(853)	(613)	(478)
25th percentile	0	0	0	0	3	14	28
50th percentile	0	0	3	16	41	118	151
75th percentile	2	11	44	101	187	434	569
90th percentile	21	64	176	320	502	804	1178
Women	(288)	(589)	(822)	(903)	(693)	(515)	(485)
25th percentile	0	0	0	0	0	0	0
50th percentile	0	0	0	0	0	4	24
75th percentile	0	0	0	10	33	87	123
90th percentile	4	9	23	66	140	310	362

The number of patients in each group is in parentheses.

It can be seen that a zero calcium score in a younger patient may not necessarily mean that that patient sits in the lowest risk group for age and sex. For example, a zero calcium score for women between 35 and 39 means that, as they age, they could eventually end up in the 25th, 50th or even the 75th percentile for age and sex *(see rectangle on chart)*. In this situation adding in fine slice assessment down to 0.6mm allows improved evaluation by potentially altering where that patient may fit within his/her age-matched cohort. In the setting of a 35–39 year-old woman, some flecks of calcium which do not register as a full score on the Agatston score, would suggest it is possible that patient sits between the 75th and 90th percentile.

An easy example of this is to take a calcium score of 28. On its own this is not a particularly high-risk feature. It carries with it a risk of an event over the next 10 years of approximately 3.5 percent. If, however, we were to obtain a coronary calcium score of 28 in two separate individuals then the significance of that result, when percentiles are taken into account, becomes more obvious.

For a male aged between 65 and 70 years, a coronary calcium score of 28 falls within the first 25 percent for age and sex for that population. This would be considered a relatively low-risk finding and would be unlikely to have significant upward pressure on that risk based on the absolute calcium score alone. *For a female aged between 45 and 49 years,* a coronary calcium score of 28 would fall above the 90th percentile for age and sex. This is a markedly elevated coronary calcium score for age and sex and would have a significant, upward effect on the risk, as assessed by the absolute score alone[1].

So, the absolute coronary calcium score then can be viewed through the prism of the calcium score percentile for age and sex, such that an approximation to a propensity for the development of atheroma can be assessed.

So for primary prevention screening, I generally stop at a zero calcium score for men 50 years or older, and women 60 years or older[2]. For younger patients with significant risk factors, however, I will often progress to a CCTA if there are specks of calcium found on the 'fine cut' (that is 0.6mm slices) even if the Agatston Score (based on three millimetre slices) is zero[3,4].

This discussion has been concerned with traditional risk factors.

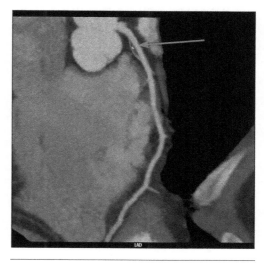

The image for this 30-year-old man with a terrible family history of premature coronary artery disease shows a small speck of calcium at the origin of the LAD (main artery down the front of the heart), although he had a zero calcium score.

This image also shows a large non-calcific plaque with the speck of calcium in the middle of it. For this case obtaining the CCTA shows the real risk for this young man. This is a high-risk plaque and without treatment would lead to this young man following the family tradition!

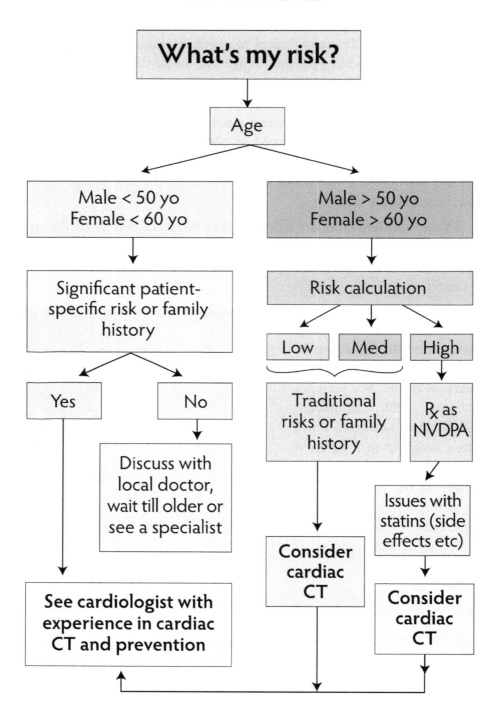

Plaque and risk

The next stage is to look at **plaque-specific** factors. A CCTA, which involves injecting contrast into a vein in the arm, will outline the details of the arteries so that the structure and characteristics of individual plaque can be more thoroughly assessed.

CHOLESTEROL-DOMINANT PLAQUE The most important issue that I now look for is cholesterol-dominant plaque within the artery.

Cholesterol-dominant plaque, or **non-calcific** plaque or **low attenuation plaque** (LAP), is the description of the build-up of lipid or fat within the plaque. The extent to which this occurs can have a significant bearing on the stability of the plaque. Our understanding around the development of plaque rupture indicates that increasing lipid content is associated with less stability and so a greater likelihood of rupture. Observational study shows that once a low attenuation plaque is greater than eight millimetres in length and two millimetres in diameter (a LAP volume greater than 20mm^3), it starts to carry a significant increased risk of event over the next few years.

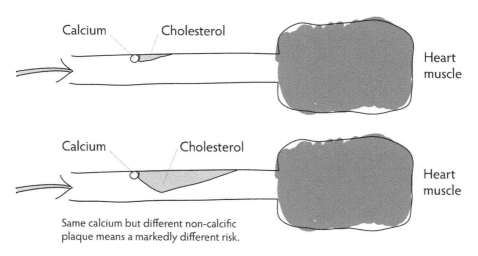

Same calcium but different non-calcific plaque means a markedly different risk.

The diagram shows two spots of calcium in an artery but they point to very different risk profiles due to the amount of associated cholesterol-laden plaque.

This is very important as it is possible to find significant low attenuation plaque in the setting of a low coronary calcium score and relatively low calcium score percentile. In this situation, the risk associated with the individual plaque becomes dominant in the future likelihood of the development of a major adverse coronary event for the individual patient. The significance of this is that, although CCS is well validated for use in risk prediction, it can dramatically underestimate risk in patients who display non-calcific plaque deposition in excess of calcium deposition. This reiterates my point that the most comprehensive assessment of the health of the arteries, if calcium is demonstrated, is the combination of both CCS and CCTA, a complete 'cardiac scan'.

REMODELLING

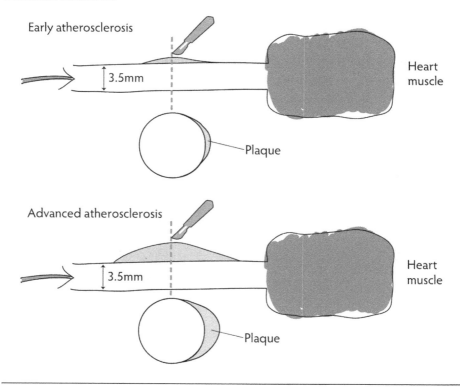

Progression of unfavourable positive remodelling

Remodelling is the process in which the vessel changes shape, enlarging to accommodate the build-up of atheroma within the artery wall. Because it can lead to enlargement, it is referred to as **positive** remodelling (although it may not be 'positive' for the patient). Initially there is no encroachment on the lumen (the inside space of the artery), yet it is a process that has been observed to carry with it a significant risk of event. Expansion changes within the artery of greater than 10 percent have been associated with rates of event of 3.5 percent in two years. This is a 15-20 percent risk over 10 years and intermediate- to high-risk of its own.

Significant fatty or low attenuation plaque (greater than 8mm x 2mm), together with unfavourable remodelling, has been observed to be associated with event rates of over 20 percent in two years. This is a 100 percent rate over 10 years and is a very, very high-risk feature.

STENOSIS A further plaque-related feature that warrants assessment in risk evaluation is stenosis or **narrowing.** There is good data suggesting that if there were a narrowing of greater than 50 percent, then the particular plaque involved could have event rates of over five percent per annum. Over 10 years this would be a 50 percent event rate and, of its own, a high- to very high-risk feature.*

SITE or LOCATION Lastly, the location of a high-risk plaque is important to factor into a risk assessment. This is common sense but is also backed by data. This supports the premise that the more proximal a ruptured plaque that gives rise to an event is, then the worse the outcome; the more distal and the smaller amount of myocardium at risk, then the better the prognosis.

IMPORTANT POINTS

- Traditional and plaque-specific risk features should be used in combination.

- Coronary calcium scoring is a very powerful negative predictive test.

- Calcium build-up in arteries increases with age.

- Some patients, particularly young ones, may have their risk underestimated by CCS alone. However, thinner slices can pick up calcium in younger patients.

- The CCS percentile for sex and age is useful in risk stratification.

- A high measure of calcium for age and sex increases risk further.

- Features of the plaque that can be considered in relation to increased risk are:

  » the extent to which the plaque is cholesterol-dominant;

  » the extent to which the artery has been remodelled (expanded unfavourably);

  » the extent to which the plaque has caused stenosis (narrowing) within the artery, and

  » the site of plaque.

[1]   Budoff MJ, Shaw LJ, Liu ST, et al. Long-term prognosis associated with coronary calcification: observations from a registry of 25,253 patients. J Am Coll Cardiol 2007;49:1860-70.

[2]   Georgiou D, Budoff MJ, Kaufer E, Kennedy JM, Lu B, Brundage BH. Screening patients with chest pain in the emergency department using electron beam tomography: a follow-up study. J Am Coll Cardiol 2001;38:105-10.

[3]   Budoff MJ, Nasir K, McClelland RL, et al. Coronary calcium predicts events better with absolute calcium scores than age-sex-race/ethnicity percentiles: MESA (Multi-Ethnic Study of Atherosclerosis). J Am Coll Cardiol 2009;53:345-52.

[4]   Latif MA, Budoff MJ. Role of CT angiography for detection of coronary atherosclerosis. Expert Rev Cardiovasc Ther 2014;12:373-82.

[5]   Cho I, Chang H-J, Sung JM, et al. Coronary computed tomographic angiography and risk of all-cause mortality and non-fatal myocardial infarction in subjects without chest pain syndrome from the CONFIRM Registry (COronary CT Angiography EvaluatioN for Clinical Outcomes: an InteRnational Multicenter Registry). Circulation 2012:CIRCULATIONAHA. 111.081380.

[6]   Al-Mallah MH, Qureshi W, Lin FY, et al. Does coronary CT angiography improve risk stratification over coronary calcium scoring in symptomatic patients with suspected coronary artery disease? Results from the prospective multicenter international CONFIRM registry. European Heart Journal-Cardiovascular Imaging 2014;15:267-74.

[7]   Agatston AS, Janowitz WR, Hildner FJ, Zusmer NR, Viamonte JM, Detrano R. Quantification of coronary artery calcium using ultrafast computed tomography. J Am Coll Cardiol 1990;15:827-32.

[8]   Aslam A, Khokhar US, Chaudhry A, et al. Assessment of isotropic calcium using 0.5-mm reconstructions from 320-row CT data sets identifies more patients with non- zero Agatston score and more subclinical atherosclerosis than standard 3.0- mm coronary artery calcium scan and CT angiography. Journal of cardiovascular computed tomography 2014;8:58-66.

[9]   Raggi P, Gongora MC, Gopal A, Callister TQ, Budoff M, Shaw LJ. Coronary artery calcium to predict all-cause mortality in elderly men and women. J Am Coll Cardiol 2008;52:17-23.

[10] Raggi P, Cooil B, Callister TQ. Use of electron beam tomography data to develop models for prediction of hard coronary events. Am Heart J;141:375-82.

[11] Budoff MJ, Hokanson JE, Nasir K, et al. Progression of coronary artery calcium predicts all-cause mortality. JACC: Cardiovascular Imaging 2010;3:1229-36.

---

* The calculation of probability is more complicated than this, please forgive artistic licence to emphasize the point. The actual calculation would be: 80% chance per two years of not having an event, so 0.8^5 gives a rate of not having an event in 10 years of 0.33. So rate of event is 1-0.3 = 70% over 10 years, which are still very high odds!

In the next chapter we look at bringing precision to the reporting of an individual's risk stratification.

Chapter 9 -
Reporting a clear message

> the importance of the report

Currently, there are two major data sets relating to cardiac CT. The first outlines coronary calcium scoring and strongly supports the use of calcium as a marker for cardiovascular risk. The second set relates to the reliability of CT coronary angiography for an **anatomical** or structural description of the coronary arteries.

The Society of Cardiac Computed Tomography, in the latter part of 2014, released its guidelines for interpretation and reporting CCTA[1]. This document focussed predominantly on the interpretation of CT coronary angiography and on the description around a detailed reproducible format of reporting for the findings anatomically. Although calcium scoring is mentioned, there is no comment regarding risk interpretation in the reporting guidelines.

In my practice, I review a patient who, if indicated, is then prepared for a cardiac CT with appropriate heart-rate-regulating medication. I review that patient's scan so that I have a feel for the state of the arteries. This means that when I consult with the patient after the scan, I have the benefit of seeing, if you like, the picture of that person's heart.

I believe a picture 'is worth a thousand words'. **The opportunity to make a risk assessment, having looked at the health of someone's arteries, is an extraordinary opportunity and, to my way of thinking, is without question, beneficial.** This is because it is very hard to report the anatomical findings within an artery and expect the referring doctor, who may not necessarily have expertise in cardiac CT imaging, to understand what the anatomical description means in regard to risk.

Let me clarify this with an example. A report may read:

"calcific and non-calcific plaque and changes consistent with early remodelling demonstrated in the proximal left anterior descending with no evidence of flow limitation".

This anatomical description could be absolutely correct. However, unless the doctor who will be acting on that report understands exactly what this anatomical description means, the doctor will not be able to put it into an appropriate context for risk modification for that patient. If the doctor reads *"no evidence of flow limitation"* and mistakenly considers this reassuring, then he or she would be wrong and the patient may be under-treated for future cardiovascular risk.

The unit I work within reports according to the guidelines of the SCCT. It has been my observation, however, that we do not report in a way that necessarily allows a specialist without expertise in cardiac CT imaging, or a general practitioner who has referred a patient for risk stratification, to have an appropriate grasp of the risk that the patient may actually carry, based on the scan features alone.

Following are some excerpts from reports that have been generated from our unit and sent back to the referring doctor; I have been a co-reporter. I offer them to show that, for a medical practitioner not fully aware of all the subtleties related to risk within calcium scoring and CT coronary angiography, these reports do not provide clear guidance for risk management in the individual patient. Below each report I have added a comment to aid your understanding.

REPORT: *Heavy calcification over proximal coronary arteries, precluding further assessment with CT coronary angiography. Agatston score 1649.5*

COMMENT: This is a very high coronary calcium score and would suggest high- to very high-risk of a MACE.

REPORT: *Moderate plaque burden. Areas of mild to moderate stenosis in the LAD. A severe stenosis in the LAD could not be excluded. Functional/clinical correlation suggested if clinically indicated.*

COMMENT: It is hard to tell what sort of risk this patient carries. Is it mild to moderate? It is almost certainly increased but it's not easy to know for someone unfamiliar with the terminology and technology. The features would suggest high- to very high-risk of a MACE.

REPORT: *Eccentric mixed plaque in the distal left main / proximal LAD causing <50% luminal narrowing. There is no other visible disease. Although the actual volume of disease is small, placing the patient between the 25-50th percentiles for age and gender, the location of disease is concerning. Aggressive risk management is recommended.*

COMMENT: This is the beginnings of a risk comment, although risk is not actually mentioned. Suggesting aggressive risk management probably means it looks pretty high risk on the scan but what is 'aggressive risk management'? Is it statin therapy to target? What if statin is not tolerated? Does the patient need to lose weight? Exercise? Is it to treat diabetes or pre-diabetes? Is dialysis/plasmaporesis required to remove cholesterol from the blood stream? Is it a stent? Is it cardiac surgery? Is it enrolment in a trial for one of the new lipid-lowering agents? Does it include family screening?

The point is that the report of a scan, often generated by a reporting specialist(s) who may not have seen or spoken to the patient, cannot of its own dictate how a patient is managed. Surely, it is better to give the referring clinician a clearer indication of the risk that may be suggested by the scan, and then let the practitioner decide what management is required, based on a comprehensive understanding of the patient's clinical details.

From this background, with a realisation that cardiac CT imaging (combining CCS and CCTA) offers an insight into the health of the arteries and so potentially provides information that could improve risk management for that individual patient into the future, I realised that reports that gave risk guidance to the referring doctor could be beneficial for patient care.

As I have mentioned earlier, the language that we use around cardiovascular risk in medicine is low, intermediate and high risk of a major adverse coronary event. Low risk is up to 10 percent risk of an event in 10 years; high risk is greater than a 20 percent risk of an event in 10 years, and intermediate risk is in between.

From a practical perspective, I believe that if we can produce reports from cardiac CT imaging which use this sort of language, then the information will be accessible and relatable to the referring doctor, regardless of whether or not that practitioner has expertise in cardiac CT imaging. This would then benefit the patient.

The C-PLUSS Model for risk evaluation

Using the features that I look for *(as outlined in the previous chapter)*, I use a simple acronym that allows me to be more precise in reporting risk evaluation:

I report cardiac CT in terms of anatomy using the standard convention and in keeping with

C-PLUSS	
C	Calcium score
P	calcium score Percentile
L	Low attenuation plaque
U	Unfavourable positive remodelling
S	Stenosis
S	Site (or location) of plaque

the SCCT guidelines. I add the C-PLUSS comment when speaking with patients and also in my explanation back to the general practitioner who will be caring for the patient into the future. In the following example, you will see that the features are described as "been observed to be associated with". This is a deliberate use of language, as the basis of the C-PLUSS model is derived from observational studies.

Standard Report

The CCS is 550 distributed over the left main (32), the LAD (294), the RCA (156) and Cx (68). There is proximal and mid-LAD mixed plaque demonstrating positive remodelling with stenosis up to 50%. There is proximal Cx mixed plaque, less than 20%. There is proximal RCA mixed plaque, with positive remodelling less than 50% stenosis and mixed plaque at the origin of the PDA less than 20%.

Three vessel disease without flow limitation.

Risk Comment

The CCS is high (550). This has been observed to be linked to risk of a MACE of 10 to 15% in 10 years. The CCS percentile is >75. This would suggest an increase in risk based on CCS alone by severalfold, and carry an increased lifetime risk.

Presence of significant non-calcific plaque burden, with associated unfavourable positive remodelling, has been observed to be associated with event rates up to 20% in 2 years. This is a very high-risk feature.

The location of disease in the Left Main, proximal LAD, Cx and RCA is concerning due to the territory potentially affected by an event.

The features of this cardiac CT study have been observed to be associated with high to very high (>>20% risk in 10 y) CV risk. This information should be combined with an evaluation of the patient's other CV risk factors for a comprehensive risk profile to help in guiding further management.

The report deliberately avoids vague terms such as "aggressive treatment" and describes risk features that are present at the time of scanning, without comment on other traditional risk factors. It is up to the referring doctor to take the cardiac scan information and apply it to the patient as appropriate.

To the average reader, all this may seem hard work and too complicated to worry about. The reason I include it, however, is for you. If you do choose to undertake cardiac CT scanning to evaluate your own risk, particularly if you have invested your own money to do so, I think you will want to make sure the report you receive is what you paid for and something from which you will actually benefit. So, feel free to ask your doctor and/or the provider of the scan if a <u>structured risk comment</u> is being used in the reports. If not, you know where to direct them. I have included in the appendix a copy of a paper I co-authored on this topic in Cardiology Today. It provides more detail and supporting references.

IMPORTANT POINTS

- Describing what is there is the anatomy.
- Interpreting the anatomy is the risk.
- Understanding the patient is clinical.
- Combining the anatomy with risk and the clinical picture gives management.

[1]   Leipsic J, Abbara S, Achenbach S, et al. SCCT guidelines for the interpretation and reporting of coronary CT angiography: A report of the Society of Cardiovascular Computed Tomography Guidelines Committee. Journal of cardiovascular computed tomography;8:342-58.

The next chapter explains why the news is always good news.

Chapter 10 -
Planning your own heart attack (NOT!)

> making your own plans:

- do you want to be forewarned and prepared?

> what's the alternative?

By now you will have learnt a little bit about the heart and the coronary arteries. You now know about atherosclerotic plaque, how it can be calcific dominant or 'cholesterol' or non-calcific dominant, and how its build-up can be patchy through the arteries.

You understand that traditional risk factors are important but still don't tell you what is going on in **your** arteries. Eating a 'healthy diet', exercising, not being overweight are all good things but they do not necessarily protect you. They only help predict risk in a population of individuals with the same characteristics.

You also realise that elevated cholesterol isn't always associated with problems in the arteries. You may be in the position of wanting to know if a statin that has been recommended for you is really required based on what is going on in **your** arteries.

You are aware of the reassurance of a zero coronary calcium score (for men over 50 and women over 60 years of age) and how, if there is calcium present in the arteries, undertaking CCTA will provide the most accurate way to assess plaque specific characteristics. You know that combining the calcium score with the calcium score percentile, then looking at plaque specific characteristics will provide the most information to make a risk assessment from the cardiac CT scan. This needs to be integrated with the individual's clinical characteristics. Treatment is then based on the combination of the patient's traditional risk features and the plaque-specific risk features.

I have employed this approach with 2500-3000 patients over the past five years. To date, I have not had a single out-of-hospital cardiac arrest in the patients who have remained on the prescribed medication and continued with appropriate follow up.

You have some choice in this. The more informed you are, the better the choices you can make.

The 2013 ACC/AHA (American College of Cardiology/American Heart Association) guideline on the assessment of cardiovascular risk covers the topic of traditional risk factors comprehensively. That recommendation says that adults between 20 and 79 years of age should be evaluated every four years using traditional risk factors. If their 10 year risk is greater than 7.5 percent then they should be evaluated into a high-risk category; if their risk is less than 7.5 percent, then a 30 year lifetime risk can be evaluated[1].

In Australia, we use the Australian Cardiovascular Risk Disease Calculator which includes age, sex, total cholesterol level, HDL cholesterol, smoking status, diabetes status and presence of left ventricular hypertrophy (which is thickening of the heart muscle) on ECG. *(http://www.cvdcheck. org.au/)* Interestingly, neither the American nor Australian traditional risk factor calculators include family history, diet, exercise, weight nor waist-to-hip ratio. Both American and Australian approaches are based on populations and both have the inherent limitations of that approach. **They are excellent for predicting within a population but not for the individual.**

The thrust of this book is to raise awareness around the possibility of using cardiac CT imaging as a way to look at a population and find the *individuals* within that population who would be at higher or lower risk than the average of that population.

My approach is to routinely scan men at 50 years of age and women at 60 years of age, as it tends to be the following 10 to 15 years when the majority of unexpected cardiac events occur in the intermediate-risk population. My observation is that there tends to be family clusters and so I lower the 50/60 age if there is a significant family history of premature coronary artery disease, particularly if associated with unfavourable risk markers. I consider scanning the individual patient 5 to 10 years earlier than the family's first event to ensure we are ahead of the game. The other situation in which I consider earlier scanning for risk is if there are significant traditional risks (for example, very high cholesterol, obesity, pre-diabetes, diabetes, high blood pressure, being a smoker) that could mean a young patient may be carrying a significant likelihood of a heart attack. The timing of this, I believe, is a specialist area and would warrant the patient seeing a cardiologist with an interest in cardiac CT imaging and prevention. This would ensure the most appropriate use of the technology and the best possible interpretation of the results.

In general, I tend to be more interested in the lipid profile (cholesterol levels and different lipoprotein levels) *after* the scan results, as this shows what is going on in the arteries and is our guide to intervention. Lipid issues should be discussed with someone who has interest and knowledge in the field.

Before undertaking any screening, it is important for a patient to be aware that knock-on effects may result from the scan. I make a point of explaining to patients that because insurance companies do not have a clear understanding of where this technology fits, an abnormality could have a detrimental impact on a person's ability to obtain re-insurance. To that end, I recommend that patients who are about to undergo cardiac CT imaging for risk stratification speak with their insurance brokers to obtain information around what impact the findings of the scan may have on their insurance. Not only does this forewarn them but it also allows them to put appropriate guaranteed, renewable insurance in place, if necessary. I do not try to cover the detail of insurance with patients, as it is not my area of expertise, but I do feel an obligation to raise it as an issue that needs to be considered before obtaining information which would need to be considered as part of a full disclosure.

Similarly, there are some occupations in which interpretation of findings related to atheroma build-up on cardiac CT scan could have an untoward effect on accreditation, certification or licensing. For example, the finding of a significant atheroma burden in a commercial pilot could well lead to a request for further testing or evaluation by the licensing board. To be aware of these issues prior to undertaking the initial investigation is nothing more than being prepared.

However, one should not lose sight of the main objective here. Not checking your heart because of possible problems with insurance or licensing could result in your paperwork being in order but you are no longer here!

Lastly, in relation to the evaluation of chest pain (particularly sudden onset [A&E-type] chest pain which arises as a symptom occurring *de novo*), my strong recommendation is to explore whether the particular situation is one that could be evaluated using cardiac CT imaging, so that not only a diagnosis of anatomical significance is provided *(Is there a narrowing or not?)* but also information that would yield prognostic information *(Is there a significant atheroma burden that could mean increased risk of a heart attack in the future?)*.

Whatever the news, it's good news

I have had patients and even colleagues say to me they just don't want to know what's going on with their heart. They don't want to know in case it is bad news. Well, I can understand this as a knee-jerk response but really it is ostrich behaviour. Sticking your head in the sand is not going to solve anything, nor allow sensible planning, whatever the situation may be. I say to these 'ostriches', "Do you have your car serviced? If you do, why?" The choice between finding out about brakes that may fail during a scheduled service or on a drive during a family holiday is a no-brainer. The chance to find out about potential problems can provide confronting information but what's the alternative?

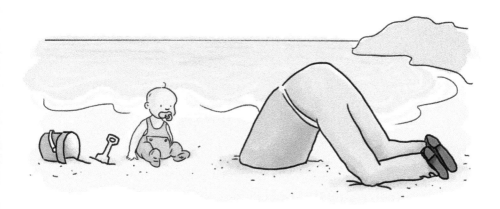

There are only fours ways to diagnose coronary artery plaque:

1) At the time of autopsy. *Too late.*

2) In the back of an ambulance on the way to hospital. *Still too late.*

3) With chest pain and shortness of breath. *Late in the process.*

4) Cardiac CT imaging – **before a problem has occurred.**

How would you want to find out?

Doctors have told me that they have had patients with high-risk findings on their scan who then suffer because of anxiety created by the findings. In my experience, this is very uncommon. I make a particular point of explaining to patients about to undergo the scan that "whatever the result, it will be helpful information". My experience is that a clear discussion with education and expectations prior to and support after the test means the results of the scan are dealt with objectively, expending minimal emotional energy. Some patients will have an anxiety disorder which needs treatment anyway and, if it weren't the scan result, it would be something else causing concern. And sure, some doctors could learn to improve their delivery. Either way, this should not detract from the big picture.

*If the scan shows
low-risk features – great!*

Off you go.

*If the scan shows
high-risk features – great!*

*This is what we are going
to do to reduce that risk...*

Ultimately, individuals will deal with situations differently and sometimes there is little that can be done to change that. My feeling and experience, however, is that for the vast majority of patients, dealing with the facts in a sensible, balanced way makes for good sense and good medicine.

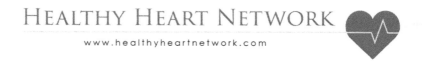

THE ULTIMATE MEMBERSHIP TO STAYING HEALTHY AND LIVING LONGER...

HEALTHY HEART NETWORK

www.healthyheartnetwork.com

Plan your heart attack (NOT!)

- **I recommend screening:** at 50 years of age for men unless there is a significant risk factor at play and, for women, as they tend to follow men's risk by about 10 years, at 60, again unless other risk factors come into play.

- You will need to **discuss screening with your regular doctor.** The doctor may not be familiar enough with the technology to answer all your questions, or may not be comfortable with requesting the test through lack of experience with it. You may need to see a cardiologist with an interest in the area, someone like me, who can best assess your needs and make the appropriate arrangements for heart rate control which is required for optimal scanning. I see many patients in this capacity.

- You will need to find a centre that has the **right equipment**: a minimum of a 64 slice CT scanner. Your referring doctor should know this.

- It is best to have a centre that has **both a radiologist and a cardiologist** onsite, as both bring different skills to acquiring the test and its quality.

- That centre also needs to have **experience** obtaining the images with **good image quality** and **low radiation doses.** Have your scan done at a high-volume centre that concentrates on best image quality at lowest achievable radiation doses. Again, your referring doctor should know this.

- Once you have had the scan, then it needs to be **reported** in a way that relates to the risk features demonstrated. I recommend the C-PLUSS approach in addition to the report fulfilling the SCCT guidelines.

- The results of the scan then need to be discussed with you and a **plan for future management** made. Some local doctors may have the experience to deal with this, particularly if the findings are straightforward; some won't. I see it as a very important part of the care I provide for a patient through the screening process.

- If your results are high- to very high-risk, **see a cardiologist.**

Remember, whatever the result, it's GREAT.

IMPORTANT POINTS

- For the reader who is the patient ...

  » You have a choice in your care and the ongoing management of your situation.

  » Gather as much information as possible.

  » Understand the risk and benefits **for you!**

  » Deal with doctors or specialists with cardiac CT experience.

  » I wish you all the best!

[1]   *Eckel RH, Jakicic JM, Ard JD, et al. 2013 AHA/ACC Guideline on Lifestyle Management to Reduce Cardiovascular Risk: A Report of the American College of Cardiology/American Heart Association Task Force on Practice Guidelines. Circulation 2014;129:S76-S99.*

The next chapter encourages you to join the conversation and be part of changing medical practice.

Testimonial

I am 52 years of age, work in an office position and have always struggled with my weight. That, combined with a family history of heart disease, has worried me that I could die prematurely of a heart-related condition. In recent years I have managed to drop my weight by about 28kg (adopting a low carbohydrate eating plan for some of this weight loss) and have incorporated exercise into my daily routine. However, I always had in the back of my mind that I still could have a high risk of suffering a heart attack.

I visited my GP in January 2015 for a general check-up and discussed the cardiac CT scanning idea with her. My GP ran the online cardiovascular disease risk calculator which resulted in my having a one percent risk of heart attack but, because of the family history, we discussed that cardiac CT scanning would be a positive thing for me to do. I had read about it before and had always managed to find an excuse not to go through with it; this year something made me decide that I had to do it.

I made the appointment with Dr Bishop and went along for my routine blood tests beforehand. I had thought for a while that I probably should have been taking medication to lower my cholesterol although, when I had been to another GP two years previously, I was told that because I had no other symptoms, it was probably not necessary. After I received my blood test results my cholesterol, which has see-sawed over the last few years, had gone up to 6.1, so I knew that I needed to finally do something about it.

My husband came along with me to my first appointment to see Warrick Bishop and, by the end of the consultation, we had both decided to undergo the cardiac CT testing. We agreed with Dr Bishop that it would be a win-win situation to find out our risk factors and go on to medication if necessary.

I was hoping for a miracle; I hoped that I had been worrying for nothing. My husband was sceptical that it was going to be worth it.

A couple of weeks after our scans, at our follow-up appointment with Dr Bishop, my worst fears were realised. Dr Bishop explained what he had seen from my results: I had a substantial build-up of cholesterol in my arteries and my risk of heart attack was extremely high. If left untreated, I stood a high chance of having an "episode" as he put it within five years. I needed to go on to a very strong dose of cholesterol-lowering medication immediately, and he wanted to follow up with me within three months to see if the medication was making a difference. Needless to say it was a big wake-up call for me. My husband, on the other hand, had great results: no build up in his arteries and no need for medication at that time.

I have been on medication to lower my cholesterol now for three months, and after having another series of more investigative blood tests, at my latest visit Dr Bishop told me my cholesterol has dropped to 4.1. Dr Bishop is happy with my results and does not want to see me for 12 months.

I will need to continue with my medication for the rest of my life but considering what could have happened if I had continued blindly along the road on which I was headed, it may be have been a very different story.

To say that cardiac CT scanning has been a life saving experience for me is an understatement. If I had continued to put my head in the sand and not had the scan, who knows what may have happened. I am not out of the woods but am now more aware that, should I experience any symptoms of heart attack, I need to act on them quickly. It could be the difference between life and death.

I am extremely glad and very fortunate that this testing was available for my husband and me, and I extend my thanks to Dr Bishop for his encouragement and belief in this procedure.

Caroline Hardin

What has this all been for? Prevention is better than cure.

'Prevention is better than cure' and Dr Warrick Bishop's book illustrates how our patients can prevent a heart attack. This comprehensive book will not only serve as a wake-up call for many people, but also save lives.

Dr Bishop has managed to make a complicated subject easy to understand for everyone, with descriptive examples and illustrations. I will certainly be recommending this book to my patients.

Karam Kostner

Associate Professor of Medicine,
University of Queensland
and Director of Cardiology,
Mater Hospital
Brisbane, Queensland, Australia

Dr Karam Kostner's clinical interest is preventative cardiology and lipid disorders. He has also been actively involved in cardiovascular research for 15 years, mainly in the area of lipoproteins, lipid lowering and atherosclerosis.

Having published approximately 90 peer reviewed papers, four book chapters and several review articles and editorials, Dr Kostner has also given numerous invited lectures at cardiovascular meetings. He is secretary of the Cardiac Society of Australia and NZ, Queensland branch, having also been president. He is an editorial board member and section editor of the European Journal of Clinical Investigation, and a regular reviewer for many journals, as well as being a NHMRC Grant Reviewer. Dr Koster has also organised or been on the committee of several national and international conferences.

Chapter 11 -
The future

IN THIS CHAPTER WE LOOK AT

> beginning a conversation that will encourage:

  - the widespread use of cardiac CT imaging so that it will be included in public health policy

  - ongoing research into understanding, treatment and management of coronary artery disease

  - government and regulatory bodies to reconsider their approach to proactive lessening of risk

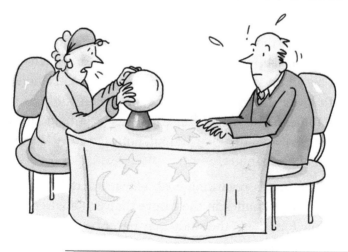

"It's telling me that a cardiac CT will do a better job of predicting your future!"

My hope from this book is to begin a conversation which ultimately increases utilisation of cardiac CT imaging, in combination with other risk factor evaluation, in order to improve primary prevention for coronary artery disease.

My vision is that imaging will be incorporated into a more holistic approach, thus improving the way we deal with the potential risk many individuals carry in regard to coronary artery disease. As this technology becomes more familiar to the community, then its use could be at the coalface for general practitioners who are, by virtue of their position in providing medical care, the custodians of preventative medicine.

Cardiac CT imaging could become the preferred tool of risk assessment for general practitioners in a way that allows the technology to appropriately guide intervention or allows a choice regarding a modified approach in an individual patient. However, until clear-cut guidelines are established, it may be that specialist involvement will be important for the most appropriate use of the technology.

As we are comfortable with mammography for breast screening, pap smears for population screening, measuring cholesterol levels and blood sugar levels, my hope is that we will see cardiac CT imaging as one of the tools available for widespread implementation in public policy.

My hope also is that there is recognition of imaging findings to help guide government-supported statin prescription, which currently in Australia is based on traditional criteria alone. This excludes a group of patients with lower intermediate-risk factor profile but high-risk features on cardiac CT imaging. It makes sense to focus treatment on what is going on in the arteries of an individual patient, not what **may** be going on in the arteries based on probability.

There will be issues regarding cost, efficacy and appropriateness. Of course, there will be studies in the future that will answer some of these questions, while for others, the study may never be done.

Widespread public screening presents the opportunity to evaluate the state of an individual person's arteries and make appropriate decisions, which are particular and specific for that individual. My feeling is it should not rely on the population in which the person sits statistically to decide the care; cardiac CT imaging allows us to be more precise than that.

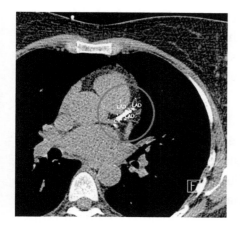

An individual who has 'a lot' of calcium in the arteries in both absolute terms, and in age and sex terms.

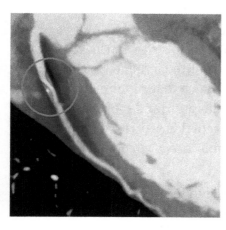

An example in which there is little calcium but considerable non-calcific (cholesterol-rich) plaque. A single plaque in the proximal LAD that leads to a MACE is 'affectionately' known as a 'widow maker'.

The future may look at repeat scanning as an appropriate tool to assess intervention. Although the current data is not clear cut, there is some research to support it[1]. In my practice, there are specific situations in which I think it is appropriate and, at this stage, it is a management strategy that is best left to specialist interpretation.

As the use of imaging the coronary arteries increases, there is no doubt in my mind that improved understanding of the underlying process of coronary atheroma will develop. In the simplest of terms, we see situations when there is a significant widespread presence of atheroma in the arteries and this is manifest with a significant calcium burden, reflective of the process of atheroma accumulation within the arteries. At the same time, however, imaging clearly demonstrates situations when minimal calcium is deposited within the arteries in the setting of significant build-up of cholesterol.

The more we image these two different ends of the spectrum and the more data we collect around these situations, the better will be our understanding and, therefore, our management into the future. We may start to be able to predict an individual's propensity to form one type of plaque or the other. One day we may even be able to predict at what location in the artery plaque is likely to occur. Wouldn't that be amazing? Only time and continued observation will facilitate this process.

Cardiac CT imaging also demonstrates situations when only one plaque exists within the entire coronary circulation. However, the location of that plaque (for example in the proximal part of the left anterior descending artery, also known as a 'widow maker') is such that rupture of that plaque can be catastrophic. I have searched the literature and spoken with experts from all over the world for an explanation of this process. I have not been able to find a good explanation, and certainly no way to predict its presence – without imaging.

My feeling is that it is probably related to local shear stress within the artery as a consequence of the path the LAD takes over the fibrous ring that separates the top part of the heart (atria) from the bottom part of the heart (ventricles). With each contraction of the heart, there is a point above the fibrous ring where the artery remains relatively fixed compared with the artery running over the ventricle. The junction of the moving and relatively fixed parts of the LAD creates a hinge point that can be subject to local stress, causing wear and tear. The consequence of this wear and tear is the development of a localised plaque. This doesn't occur in everyone thankfully, and is probably related to specific features of the path which the LAD takes. This might be a little like a scenario in which some people with knock knees develop arthritis. Some people with bow knees get arthritis.

Yet most people with straight legs probably won't have arthritis of their knees. With time and greater understanding, we may be advocating treatment of a single plaque well before an event occurs. (There is some research looking into this.)

Localised plaque is challenging. There are occasions when I have recommended that a patient take statin and aspirin for a single high-risk plaque. The plaque may be no more than 15mm in length, so the patient is going to be taking 'lifelong' treatment for one small but significant spot of cholesterol build-up. It almost seems out of proportion that a person will take a medication that will inevitably find its way through every organ of his body in order to address a single small patch of atheroma. Unfortunately, this is the best we have at the moment.

BUT ... What if, in the future, we developed antibodies which are specific to the mechanisms behind plaque development? Could we inject a serum of antibodies that would arrest the progression of plaque formation *in situ?* If it worked for a single plaque, could it work for more extensive disease? What if we could develop nano technology that could target the plaque and remove the debris and cholesterol, leaving a safe but tiny scar in the artery? What a thought: a simple injection or course of injections, to arrest the process that currently rates as the leading cause of death in Western countries! Or, it may be that we observe and understand that early stenting of a high risk, single plaque positively affects the outcome. Whichever way medical technology develops, although coronary artery disease is the single most studied human condition, we are at the beginning of those processes of observation and understanding and will have to wait until the future unveils more clarity.

Moving on

Let's not get ahead of ourselves, as exciting as the prospect might be. There are issues that can and should be addressed now. The experience of our friend, Bill, from earlier in the book, represents an excellent example of how our current approach to atheroma burden and its management requires realignment. This realignment is not only within the medical area but also within the greater community and, for this particular case, specifically within the insurance industry.

Bill's plight is representative of a very significant point: that knowing the health of one's arteries and acting accordingly is far better than having no idea and responding to disaster. **The sooner insurance companies can get their heads around this and *not* penalise patients who proactively seek to maximise their future cardiac risk management, the better.** I would suggest that the same companies would do well to realise that the stress tests they have relied on for years are no longer the best tool available for defining risk. It is time to move with the changes in technology and the benefit of improved risk modelling, so that cheaper premiums, but most importantly better health outcomes, are available for everyone.

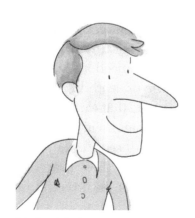

So, remember Bill, who, in the context of a borderline family history of MACE, requested cardiac CT imaging at the age of 48. Scanning was undertaken and it demonstrated a surprisingly high coronary calcium score, in fact, above the 90th percentile for age and sex. CCTA demonstrated high- to very high-risk features with possible flow limitation of the circumflex artery. His stress test at the time was negative for flow limitation. Bill, after also undergoing screening bloods for high-risk factors, ended up taking aspirin, statin, nicotinic acid (he had a low HDL cholesterol and a high lipoprotein a), ACE inhibitor, vitamin D and fish oil. He undertakes very regular exercise; his exercise capacity is such that he has trained for and completed the equivalent of an Hawaiian Ironman event. He also keeps an eye on a reduced carbohydrate eating guideline. As he did not tolerate statin well, he was on a very low dose every second or third day.

In the setting of full disclosure, Bill notified his insurance company of the findings of his cardiac CT scan. This lead to his insurance company not re-negotiating his policies. He was 'pinned down' by being proactive and looking after himself. It resulted in more restrictions and more focus on his lipid profile, which interestingly had never been that much of a problem. This response could only be described as disappointing.

The reality is that his risk, post-scan, had been more than halved with education and preventative strategies, yet his insurance company responded rigidly. It refused any re-negotiation of his policy. This is not only the wrong way around but sends the wrong message to an individual who may want to be proactive in the care of his cardiovascular health. Luckily, Bill didn't think twice about what his scan may show and what his insurer may do. He realised the information, whatever it was going to be, would benefit him and his family and that there was no point keeping his insurance premiums unchanged at the risk of dropping dead prematurely.

In Bill's situation, the context of not being able to treat as we had hoped, nor achieve the desired lower lipid levels[2], we undertook stress testing as a potential indicator of progression that could lead to narrowing (this is not stress testing to define risk). Several years into Bill's on-going management plan, with on-going surveillance stress testing, we clearly demonstrated a problem. Within the week, Bill had undergone invasive coronary angiography and had a stent inserted into the proximal circumflex artery which resulted in a full re-establishment of blood flow to that area of the myocardium, with no damage to his heart. He was back at work within several days, later resumed full exercise capacity and is again working with trying to take statins at the highest possible dose that doesn't cause side-effects. We are continuing with follow-up stress testing.

All this has occurred with an inflexible and difficult response by his insurance company. Yet his management, I believe, has been a model of what can be possible if we know what is going on in the arteries and can be ahead of the game. I would argue, given his risk is now actually reduced because he was identified and treated appropriately, that his premium should have been adjusted down, not up! Imagine receiving a letter from your insurance company thanking you for being proactive and reducing your own risk – and by the way we will reduce your premium in line with this.

I've not provided an example but the same holds for licensing bodies and health checks for remote work location, fire fighters, service personnel, truck drivers and, of course, private and commercial pilots.

Change is needed – across the spectrum of related interests.

This change and the other departures considered throughout this book will be brought about by conversation followed by action. Many conversations will be had by all manner of people – specialists, GPs, patients and interested onlookers – who will share ideas, explore further and learn from one another. We will listen as well as talk and we will appreciate the difference and the opportunities. To be transformative, our conversations need to be open-ended, collaborative and reflective, and it will take time. Firstly, though, it needs a catalyst. Hence, this book, your readership and my invitation to you to be part of the conversation.

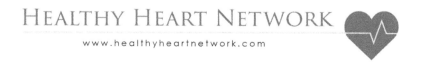

THE ULTIMATE MEMBERSHIP TO STAYING HEALTHY AND LIVING LONGER...

HEALTHY HEART NETWORK

www.healthyheartnetwork.com

IMPORTANT POINTS

- This book is the beginning of a conversation, in which you are invited to participate.

- My vision is that:

  » CT imaging will be incorporated into an holistic preventative approach to coronary artery disease;

  » imaging findings will modify government-supported statin prescriptions;

  » public screening will become widespread so that precise, individualised care will be commonplace;

  » greater understanding of the underlying process of coronary atheroma will develop leading to now-only-imagined treatment possibilities, and

  » insurance and other regulatory bodies will take a more proactive and less prescriptive view to people with plaque in their arteries.

[1] Achenbach S, Ropers D, Pohle K, et al. *Influence of Lipid-Lowering Therapy on the Progression of Coronary Artery Calcification: A Prospective Evaluation.* Circulation 2002;106:1077-82.

[2] Raggi P, Callister TQ, Shaw LJ. *Progression of coronary artery calcium and risk of first myocardial infarction in patients receiving cholesterol-lowering therapy.* Arterioscler Thromb Vasc Biol 2004;24:1272-7.

Epilogue

I have an enthusiasm about, and belief in, the technology of cardiac CT and what it can offer, tempered with an understanding of some of the hurdles preventing it from being more broadly used. From a practical as well as a logical perspective, cardiac CT imaging's contribution to improved patient care is markedly under-utilised.

The deficiency in supportive data from randomised controlled trials means that my colleagues, specifically cardiology specialists who could lead change in clinical management, are not comfortable in using the technology due to the lack of an appropriate evidence base. This scepticism can flow to general practitioners who are unlikely to unilaterally embrace a technology that does not appear to have the backing of the specialist group responsible for that area of medicine.

In focussing a spotlight on a technology that could be more widely used for the benefit of individuals and, subsequently, larger communities, I believe this book demonstrates that there is ample observational data available to support the uptake of the technology and provide guidance in the first instance. At no stage has it been my intention to diminish the importance of evidence-based medicine as the guide to how medicine decides on the direction of ongoing care. However, I believe that evidenced-based medicine should create the foundations of good medicine, not erect immoveable boundaries.

I am prepared to wear any criticism that will come my way from my evidence-based-only colleagues as, until our understanding of medicine is complete, evidence cannot provide all the answers. Nuances and variability within a circumstance, and clinical experience together with patient choice, need to be considered for good medicine to be practised.

What I also realised was that the person most interested in being aware of what is available is the patient: **YOU!** This book has been written specifically to provide information which will allow you, should you be a patient, to engage with your general practitioner and your specialist in a more detailed and robust exchange around what screening, treatment and/or management might be appropriate for you.

Criticism and controversy are healthy parts of vigorous conversation, as too, are vision, passion and an enthusiasm for possibility. If this book starts such conversation that opens doors to further evaluation, consideration and discussion – and along the way improves medicine and saves lives – then that is a good start.

Wishing you good health.

Dr Warrick Bishop

Hobart, Tasmania, Australia

Dr Bishop is available for medical and business consultancy and for speaking engagements.

Enquiries: *warrick@drwarrickbishop.com*

Visit his website *www.drwarrickbishop.com*

THE ULTIMATE MEMBERSHIP TO STAYING HEALTHY AND LIVING LONGER...

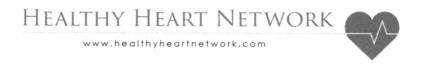

HEALTHY HEART NETWORK

www.healthyheartnetwork.com

Glossary

Acute coronary syndrome/Major Adverse Coronary Event (MACE)
the sudden development of a complete, or near complete, occlusion or blockage, of a coronary artery

> **complete blockage**
> *myocardial infarction* (*myocardial*, the heart; *infarction*, death by lack of blood flow) a complete blockage that causes the death of part of the heart muscle

> **near complete blockage**
> or 'unstable angina' puts pressure on the heart and can be the forerunner to a heart attack

Agatston Score
the standardised method of evaluating the coronary arteries for the presence of calcium. Developed by American cardiologist Arthur Agatston, the score uses three millimetre slices through the heart and then a combination of volume and density of the calcium detected to generate a 'score'.

Anatomical
relating to structure

Angina
chest pain experienced in association with reduced flow of blood to the heart. It is not a heart attack but can be an indicator of high risk.

Arteries
the vessels of the body's circulation system that carry the blood away from the heart. The aorta takes the blood from the left ventricle as the blood begins it journey around the body. Coming from the aorta as it leaves the heart are the **right coronary artery** and the **left main coronary artery.**

The left main then divides into two key arteries

> the **left anterior descending artery** (LAD) (which provides blood to the anterior surface of the heart, the area nearest the chest wall); generally the most important of the arteries, and

> **the circumflex artery** (which provides blood to the back of the heart, the area nearest the spine), as well as

> **the right coronary artery** (which provides blood to the surface of the heart the area nearest the diaphragm).

Association
connected, joined or related

Asymptomatic
producing or showing no symptoms

Atheroma
build-up of plaque within an artery

Atherosclerotic/atheromatous plaque

the build-up of cholesterol, scavenger cells, scar tissue and calcium in the wall of the artery (referred to as plaque throughout the book). The plaque can be either flow-limiting (and likely to produce symptoms) or non-flow-limiting (produces no symptoms). Also see plaque and plaque burden.

Atrium

a pre-pumping chamber (before the ventricle) on both sides of the heart

Australian absolute cardiovascular disease risk calculator

an approach to predicting risk of cardiovascular disease developed by the National Vascular Disease Prevention Alliance (NVDPA) which is an alliance of four Australian charities: Diabetes Australia, the National Heart Foundation of Australia, Kidney Health Australia and the National Stroke Foundation

Blood

the bodily fluid that conveys oxygen and nutrients to the body and removes carbon dioxide and other wastes. It carries:

platelets
small cellular fragments that are important in the forming of clots when the vascular system is damaged, e.g., they stop a cut from bleeding

red cells
the carriers of the protein, haemoglobin, which transports oxygen around the body. Red cells also remove some of the body's carbon dioxide.

Causations
factors/actions that cause the problem

Cholesterol
a lipid or fat molecule that is used as a component of cell walls and is also a precursor to synthesis of a number of hormones

Computed Tomography (CT)
see electron beam computed tomography

Coronary atheroma burden
term used, in a primary preventative setting, to describe the build-up of plaque within the arteries in a patient who is otherwise well (before the development of disease)

Coronary artery bypass grafting
major surgery that allows a 'bypassing' of the diseased section of the artery by using an alternate vessel, usually from the aorta, to supply blood to the heart

Coronary Artery Calcium (CAC)
the presence of calcium in the arteries (not quantified)
See also Coronary Calcium Score.

Coronary artery disease or heart disease
the process of atherosclerosis or plaque build-up in the artery that leads to a narrowing of the artery and reduced blood flow that produces symptoms (angina, shortness of breath, a heart attack)

Coronary Calcium Score (CCS)
the number, or score, generated when looking to use calcium as a marker of

plaque; the quantification of CAC
See also Agatston Score.

Coronary Computed Tomography Angiogram (CCTA)

the result when contrast (dye) injected into a patient's vein outlines the coronary arteries in exquisite detail, giving information about the location, the quality and nature of the plaque, the degree of stenosis and the size of the vessel affected
Often referred to as a CT coronary angiogram.

C-PLUSS

an acronym to help evaluate and report risk: C (Calcium score), P (calcium score Percentile), L (Low attention plaque), U (Unfavourable positive remodelling), S (Stenosis), S (Site of plaque)

Coronary risk

the possibility of a coronary event such as a heart attack:

low a less than 10 percent chance of a coronary event within 10 years

intermediate between 10 and 20 percent chance of a coronary event within 10 years

high a greater than 20 percent chance of a coronary event within 10 years

CT coronary angiogram

see Coronary Computed Tomography Angiogram (CCTA)

Disease

a symptom or loss of normal function

Distal

situated away from the centre

Echocardiogram (Echo)

a scan of the heart using ultrasound waves to acquire a picture, like a bat uses sonar
It gives information about the valves, the chambers of the heart and pressures within the heart.

Electrocardiogram (ECG)

a trace of the electrical activity through the heart acquired by electrodes
It shows the rhythm of the heart.
Features of the ECG can be used to infer the status of the heart muscle, such as ischaemia seen during a stress test.

Electron Beam Computed Tomography (EBCT)

X-rays are deflected at very high speed using enormous magnets to acquire images that are then reconstructed. This has given rise to the term Computed Tomography (CT).

Evidence-based medicine

the guidelines or recommendations (that help in the management of patients that are put together by specialty groups or organisations) are founded on research in an area
There are different levels of evidence based on the quality and amount of the research available.

Familial hypercholesterolaemia

a generic condition that gives rise to very elevated levels of cholesterol and is associated with a family history of premature coronary artery disease

Fluoroscopy
rapid acquisition x-ray to allow
assessment during movement

Framingham-type risk modelling
using multiple associations with observed
outcomes to predict likelihood of an event
or risk

Heart
a large muscle that pumps blood through
the body

Heart attack
not a medical expression
It is a layman's term referring to a major
heart problem. Most commonly it is a
narrowing of the coronary arteries that
can kill or requires some form of medical
intervention – medication, time in
hospital, balloons or stents, or coronary
artery bypass grafting.

Heart Foundation
a national charity dedicated to fighting
the single biggest killer of Australians,
heart disease
It funds life-saving heart research
and works to improve heart disease
prevention and care for all Australians.

Ischaemic heart disease
reduced blood supply to the heart

Invasive coronary angiogram
direct injection of contrast (dye) into the
coronary arteries by using a thin plastic
catheter (tube) that is passed from the
artery of the leg or from the artery of the
wrist to the origin of the aorta and guided
into the origin of the left main or right
coronary arteries

It gives very precise images of the lumen
or inside of the arteries (the inside of the
artery, not the wall).

Lipid tests
current testing for lipids covers total
cholesterol, triglycerides, high-density
lipoprotein, low-density lipoprotein,
non-high-density lipoprotein and total
cholesterol to HDL ratio

Lipoprotein
the carrier of cholesterol in the blood
(*lipo,* fat)

Lumen
the inside space of the artery, where the
blood flows

Macrophages
scavenger cells, important in the build-
up of plaque

**Major Adverse Coronary Event
(MACE)**
medical term for heart attack (see acute
coronary syndrome)

Myocardium
myo, muscle; *cardium,* being of the
heart, the muscle of the heart

**National Vascular Disease
Prevention Alliance (NVDPA)**
an alliance of four Australian charities:
Diabetes Australia, the National Heart
Foundation of Australia, Kidney Health
Australia and the National Stroke
Foundation

Negative predictive test
the condition is not present

Plaque
the build-up of cholesterol, scavenger cells, scar tissue and calcium in the wall of the artery (referred to as plaque throughout the book)
The plaque can be either flow-limiting (and likely to produce symptoms) or non-flow-limiting (produces no symptoms).

>   **unstable plaque** When the fibrous cap of the plaque ruptures, platelets in the blood begin to clump together to form a clot which may completely block the artery.
>   If it is a non-flow-limiting plaque, death may occur without any previous warning.

Plaque burden

>   **non-calcific/cholesterol dominant/low attenuation plaque (LAP)** the build-up of lipid or fat within the plaque, has a bearing on the stability of the plaque, generally reducing plaque stability
>
>   **calcific dominant** the presence of calcium in the plaque greater than the non-calcific component, generally associated with greater plaque stability

Premature coronary disease
suffering a MACE at less than approximately 55 years of age for a male and 60 years of age for a female

Preventative cardiology

>   **primary**
>   involves treatment of the unknown Patients do not display symptoms, yet they may be at high risk because of indicators such as cholesterol levels, high blood pressure, diabetes or smoking. It attempts to prevent the development of coronary disease in a patient who has not suffered an event but indicators suggest could be at risk.
>
>   **secondary**
>   involves treatment after diagnosis – those strategies that can be put in place because symptoms have been detected or an event, such as a heart attack, has occurred
>
>   **risk assessment**
>   **population based,** using multiple parameters (for example age, sex, blood pressure) to make an evaluation of an individual's chance of a MACE based on the observed rate of events in a population with the same parameters
>
>   **individual based,** imaging the arteries of an individual to make an assessment of the chance of a MACE based on the actual features seen within the individual's arteries
>
>   **observational data**
>   Databases have been compiled of features and factors found in individuals who have had coronary artery disease. The occurrence of those features and factors then lends weight to their being used as predictors for people before they have an event. This data is collected from a large number of patients. These factors are associations, not necessarily the cause, of the problem.

Proximal
situated nearer to the centre

Radiation
background radiation exposure of a
person over a year through incidental
exposure from things such as rocky
outcrops, electronic devices, atmospheric,
flying in commercial aircraft

**Randomised double-blind
control trial**
a trial design
The trial takes a population to be studied
and separates the population into two
groups in a random way ('randomised').
One group receives the intervention and
the other group (the 'control' group)
receives **no** intervention.
Neither group knows if it is being given
the true intervention or not (they are
'blinded') and the medical staff who
look after the subjects are not aware of
who is receiving the true intervention or
not (they are 'blind' also). This is called
'double-blind'.

Remodelling
a process in which the vessels change
shape
    positive remodelling
the vessel enlarges to accommodate
    the atheroma build-up within the
artery wall

Statins
a family of drugs that lowers cholesterol

Stenosis
narrowing (of the artery)

Stenting
a coronary artery disease intervention
In the intervention, an intravascular
device (balloon) within a wire scaffold
is inserted percutaneously (through the
skin), using similar technique to invasive
coronary angiography, and guided to the
site of a narrowing.
When the balloon is inflated, the artery
is opened and the wire scaffold remains
to keep it open; the scaffold is called
a **stent.** If a wire scaffold is not used
during a ballooning procedure, then it is
called **balloon angioplasty.**

Stress test
a functional test
It tests heart function. It involves
exercising the patient or giving the
patient medication to replicate exercise,
to try to reproduce the symptom under
investigation or unmask lack of blood
flow to the heart.

Stroke
a sudden blockage, or partial blockage, of
a blood vessel supplying the brain
    thrombo-embolic stroke
    when a clot which forms in the carotid
    arteries of the neck breaks off, travels
    to the brain circulation and lodges in
    a vessel, causing lack of blood supply
    beyond that point (*embolic:* carried
    through the blood stream)
    thrombotic stroke
    when a plaque ruptures and a clot
    forms at that site

haemorrhagic stroke
when a ruptured blood vessel in the
brain leads to bleeding into the brain

**atrial fibrillation thrombo-
embolic stroke**
when the chambers at the top of
the heart lose their synchronicity,
contraction of the atria fails, blood
pools within the atrium, a clot forms,
breaks free and lodges in a brain
artery

Troponin
a blood test used as a predictor when a
person presents with chest pain to assess
likelihood of the heart being involved

Veins
the vessels of the body's circulation
system that carry the blood **to** the heart
The blood collects into two major veins,
the superior vena cava and the inferior
vena cava, before draining into the right
atrium and then right ventricle.

Ventricle
the main compression (pumping)
chamber of the heart that pushes the
blood through the body
There is a right and left ventricle.

Acknowledgements

I would like to thank

- » my wife Mercia for her enduring patience, tolerance and understanding;
- » my other family and friends for their support and understanding;
- » my staff who are always fantastic – we all work together to make a meaningful difference in people's lives;
- » my patients who have engaged in an approach to risk management with belief and focus, with particular acknowledgement to those whose case histories and testimonies are included in the book;
- » my colleagues who have listened to me, encouraged me and tried to understand my perspective, and
- » my colleagues who have not heard me, who have dismissed my ideas and have drawn conclusions before listening; each of you has encouraged me to try to find a voice through this book.

A particular thanks goes to my collaborators, researchers and reviewers without whose help this book would still be a good idea awaiting its time:

» John North who has worked tirelessly behind the scenes to make everything happen;

» John Saul provided valuable feedback and friendship at every stage;

» Kelvin Aldred offered frank patient-specific feedback throughout;

» Alistair Begg provided collegial support and encouragement;

» John Nemarich gave valuable patient feedback;

» Michael McCarthy for GP review and feedback;

» my Dad made edits and suggestions that made it into the book;

» Uncle Rod Miller edited above and beyond the call of duty;

» Jillian Smith brought precision and attention to detail in her editing and proofreading;

» Charles Wooley was good enough to find the time for a low-carb beer and a foreword, in the midst of his very busy schedule;

» Frank Parish provided invaluable radiology expertise;

» Professor Matt Budoff, a world leader in CT imaging and prevention who gave me the belief in myself to undertake this project through his support and encouragement;

» Shane Anthony was a master of referencing;

» Karam Kostner, Gerald Watts and Daniel Friedman, colleagues who I hold in the highest regard, were good enough to find precious time in their busy schedules to offer feedback and edits;

» Cathy McAuliffe and I met through the internet. Her help with design has been fantastic and her professionalism without blemish, and

» Penny Edman, my ghost-writer, has been the best. I could not have done it without her. Her focus and enthusiasm have been undaunted, her passion such that I wonder if we are like two proud parents of the pages you have just read.

I am truly grateful for all the help and support.

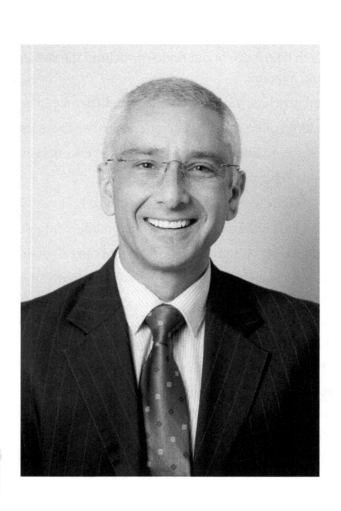

About the author

Doctor Warrick Bishop is a best selling author, keynote speaker and practising cardiologist who has a passion to help prevent heart disease on a global scale.

Warrick graduated from the University of Tasmania, School of Medicine, in 1988. He completed his advanced training in cardiology in Hobart, Tasmania, becoming a fellow of the Royal Australian College of Physicians.

A number of years ago something incredible, an amazing coincidence, happened that started Warrick on the mission to prevent heart attacks rather than try to cure them. He was driving to work one day when he stopped at a commotion by the side of the road. A fun runner had collapsed during a fun run with a heart attack. He helped in his resuscitation only to find out that had seen the very same man two years earlier and reassured him that he was fine.

Warrick had missed the chance to make a difference and it nearly cost a life!! Based on risk calculation and the best practice of the time, he shouldn't have been at high risk.....but he was!

That meant that he had reassured a patient based on treadmill testing, the best care available at the time that he was fine, only to be part of the team that resuscitated that man when he dropped dead during a running race, this was just not good enough, and he asked himself could this be done differently?

This important question started him on a journey which meant he was open to looking more closely at new and emerging technology to help in being more precise about the risk of heart attack.

It became clear to Warrick the more precise we can be in the information we have in regard to a patient's heart health and real risk of heart attack, the better we can look after that person, it seems so obvious when you say it like that, but that opportunity is still only new and not broadly utilised in the medical community.

Building on that success, Warick has decided to create a program to help people manage their risks better. It's called "The Healthy Heart Network". With The Healthy Heart Network, he can now help reduce heart disease as a major killer in the world!

Warrick holds a number professional certifications and achievements:

- First cardiologist in Tasmania with this specialist recognition in CT Cardiac Coronary Angiography
- Level B certification, with the Australian Joint Committee for CCTA
- Member of the Society of Cardiac Computed Tomography.
- Member of the Australian Atherosclerosis Society
- A participant on the panel of 'interested parties' developing a model of care and national registry for familial hypercholesterolaemia.
- Warrick is an accredited examiner for the Royal Australian College of Physicians and is regularly involved with teaching medical students and junior doctors.
- Worked with Hobart's Menzies Institute for Medical Research on projects in an affiliate capacity
- Recognised by the Medical School of the University of Tasmania with academic status.
- Member of the Clinical Issues Committee of the Australian Heart Foundation, providing input into issues of significance for the management of heart patients.

In his free time, Warrick enjoys travel and music with his wife, and he surfs and plays guitar with his children.

If you enjoyed "Know Your Real Risk Of Heart Attack" but would be interested in more information then you may also enjoy "Have You Planned Your Heart Attack" which was Dr Warrick's first book on Cardiac CT imaging and contains everything that is in "Know Your Real Risk of Heart Attack" plus more on:

- Cholesterol
- Statins
- What makes a good screening test
- Plaque formation
- Investigating chest pain
- Holistic evaluation
- Managing symptoms and prognosis
- Risk of stroke
- Chance findings
- Particular high-risk findings
- Hurdles to change
- Can we afford it?
- Appendices, published articles on nomenclature and C-PLUSS and user guide.

Find out more at : www.drwarrickbishop.com/books/

Wishing you the best information for your best health.

Dr Warrick Bishop

Printed in Australia
AUHW021448121222
372503AU00035B/81